THE TROUBLED
DREAM OF LIFE

*In Search of
a Peaceful Death*

THE TROUBLED

DREAM OF LIFE

In Search of
a Peaceful Death

DANIEL CALLAHAN

Georgetown University Press / Washington, D.C.

Georgetown University Press, Washington, D.C.

© 2000 by Georgetown University Press. All rights reserved.
Printed in the United States of America

10   9   8   7   6   5   4   2000

This volume is printed on acid-free offset book paper.

Library of Congress Cataloging-in-Publication Data
CALLAHAN, DANIEL, 1930–
THE TROUBLED DREAM OF LIFE : IN SEARCH OF A PEACEFUL
DEATH / DANIEL CALLAHAN.
P.   CM.
ORIGINALLY PUBLISHED: NEW YORK : SIMON & SCHUSTER, 1993.
INCLUDES INDEX.
ISBN 0-87840-815-0 (PAPER : ALK. PAPER)
I. DEATH.   2. TERMINAL CARE.   I. TITLE.
R726.8.C34   2000
174'.24—DC21   00-026365

ACKNOWLEDGMENTS

I long ago learned that it is perfectly possible to write a book without having another soul look at it prior to publication. I also learned that this is not wise. We profit from the counsel and criticisms of others, and that has been true with this book. A number of my friends and colleagues read draft chapters. They have improved this book greatly, even if I have not always taken their advice. Courtney Campbell has, once again, been a careful and thoughtful reader. Gilbert Meilaender not only read the manuscript but had to put up with a number of letters from me arguing about this point or that to which he had objected. He probably should have been spared such a response, but he invited it by his willingness to listen and to answer. Joseph Fins, Stephen I. Chavras, Linda Emanuel, and Norton Spritz, all physicians, provided me with a helpful combination of medical experience and ethical insight. Another physician, Eric Cassell, has been immensely helpful over the years in teaching me to understand the meaning of suffering for the sick and dying. My colleagues Willard Gaylin, Bruce Jennings, James L. Nelson, Ellen Moskowitz, and Susan Wolf each made many helpful suggestions along the way.

I was able to discuss a number of the ideas in this book with other colleagues and visitors during our daily luncheons at The Hastings Center. Darrel Amundsen gave me the benefit of his historical knowledge, always enriching. Susan Glassman gave me the help of an expert outside editorial eye. My wife, Sidney, was forced, yet again, to talk endlessly with me about topics that are not always the easiest or most pleasant for domestic conversation. Her good sense and extensive knowledge are a great marital benefit. Ellen McAvoy was, as always, indispensable in helping me prepare the manuscript. Finally, I want to thank my editor, Alice Mayhew, who has worked with me on this and earlier books. She is a splendid editor and a no less splendid friend.

The phrase in the title, "The troubled dream of life," is taken from an essay by William Hazlitt, "The Fear of Death," from his *Table Talk* (1822).

For
Alexander Morgan Capron
Eric J. Cassell
Renée C. Fox
Margaret O'Brien Steinfels
Peter Steinfels

Good friends, stimulating colleagues

CONTENTS

Introduction:

CAN DEATH BE SHAPED
TO OUR OWN ENDS?

Like any other adult with some accumulated years behind me, I have known many people who have died and are no longer part of my life. A few of those deaths are more vivid in my memory than others — in great part, I suspect, because they came to symbolize some of the many possible ways of dying. My grandmother's death in her mid-eighties, when I was about ten, remains in my imagination as a perfect kind of old-fashioned ending. She died at home in her sleep, of causes never divulged to me other than "old age," and was laid out in the living room, where neighbors, friends, and family came to pay what were called their "last respects." I do not recall any weeping or great sorrow. She had lived a long life, and her death seemed to be taken for granted. The visitors chatted and gossiped, as if it were just another social gathering of the kind she had presided over for years.

Many years later, planning a surprise visit to a sick friend, I came to his home only to discover that it was filled with people. There, in a sitting position in his bedroom, surrounded by animated friends, was his body. He had died less than an hour earlier of cancer, a death long expected. There was no weeping that time either, though he was a much-beloved person. His newly widowed wife, sensing my feeling of awkwardness, went out of her way to put me at ease: "I'm so glad you could be here, Dan. Wouldn't you like something to eat?"

I contrast those memories, benign and reassuring about death, about the way we can die, with some others. In one instance, when I was in my late teens, I knew nothing about how the person actually died, or even who had died. I was passing by a church and, my curiosity piqued by a solitary hearse outside, went inside to discover a funeral mass in progress. Other than the priest and an altar boy, not a single person was present. I wonder to this day how someone could have died so alone, even though I know that in modern life it is a common occurrence. Every few years, there is a newspaper story about Potter's Field in New York, filled with thousands of unknown dead. The memory of that lonely funeral still chills, emblematic of a life cut off from human company even as it was on its way to an even more radical separation. I am reminded of an epitaph on a gravestone reported by Nathaniel Hawthorne, of one John Treeo, who died in 1810:

> Poorly lived,
> And poorly died,
> Poorly buried,
> And no one cried.[1]

The sudden crib death of an infant son, a long, wakeful train trip at night with his coffin in the baggage car, is not easily forgotten either. Babies still die that way, and parents still cry. Then there is the long and lingering decline in hospitals of many adults I have known, including my own parents, routine enough now for the hospitals but never easily accepted by the rest of us. First there was the anxiety whether death was coming, then the certainty that it was, then the waiting. Though it did not happen to me, I have had a number of friends whose elderly parents died after an extended stay in nursing homes, long demented and cut off from human communication. They lived with the particular hell of loving their parent, wishing that parent would die, blaming themselves for having such a wish, and dutifully paying painful visits.

I cannot claim that my experience with death is anything more than average. Yet that experience, however limited, has convinced me that it is remarkably difficult to talk about death and its meaning. Odd as this may seem at a time when the subject of death has long been the routine fare of the media, talk shows, and classroom, I have told few others of my own experiences, and only a few people have told me about theirs. Or, to be more precise, we—both in my own circles and more generally—have talked about the event of death, and the process of dying, but not what we make of death itself, its human import. Death has not come out of the closet; only its foot is showing.

I say this as one whose professional life, for nearly twenty-five years, has been full of conversations and debates about death and dying. Yet, as I think back on those years, and the national debate as a whole, I am struck by a certain peculiarity, mirroring my own experience. The debate has mainly been about law, regulation, moral rules, and medical practice, and about making legal, or ethical, or medical choices about dying. It has not been about death itself, about how we should think it through in our lives. The debate is filled, to be sure, with stories and anecdotes about how people die in our day, but the main purpose of these is usually to bolster the discussion about social policy, not illuminate our personal lives. Rarely is an effort made to take the policy argument to the more troublesome depths of the place and meaning of death in human life.

That is probably not a matter for astonishment in a society more comfortable with legal than with philosophical or religious discourse, and more at ease with moral language focused on the making of decisions than with the wisdom of those decisions. To talk about death itself, and how it should find a place in our self-conception, is more troubling. It is surely unsettling in a society that has come to use the veil of pluralism to eliminate serious interchange on the deepest problems. They have been banished to the private realm, not to be let loose in the public square.

The aim of this book is, in its most modest scope, to propose what I hope are some plausible ways of bringing the legal and policy issues in the care of the dying and critically ill back into closer contact with some of the oldest questions of human existence. How might we try to think about death in our own lives? What should it mean to us, and what kind of persons should we try to become as we approach our end? How ought we to bear pain, suffering, and fear? They are questions of meaning, purpose, and character. Beyond those most private, but potent, questions are others as well, moving into different areas of our lives, individually and collectively. What kind of stance toward death should be taken by our culture—the culture that will underlie and influence our social policies and practices? I want, then, to see if I can at least stimulate a richer exchange on some old questions in the context of our more recent interest in matters of law and policy.

I have a more ambitious hope as well. I would like to persuade people that many of our problems in the care of the dying, both in public attitudes and medical practice, stem from some mistaken views of death. They are often subtle, not obvious, mistakes, of a kind easy to fall into; and into them we have fallen. For all of its great triumphs, contemporary medicine does not know what to make of death. The end of life represents a troubling, and peculiarly recent, vacuum in its thinking. Death has no well-understood place in medical theory, even if it remains omnipresent in practice. It is the enemy, standing outside the walls, to be fought and repulsed. But what is medicine to do when death finally wins? Should it understand that death must and will happen, or treat it as a temporary setback only? Medicine's own problems with death are exacerbated by the troubled perception of the public, uncertain whether death should be accepted or rejected. That public is as confused, as ambivalent, as medicine; and the two confusions work on, and influence, each other.

A major part of my more ambitious purpose is to see if we can somehow be prodded as a people to begin the work of creating a common view of death, not just choices about death, appropriate for our time, place, and society. I do not look for a rigid or a monolithic view, but at least one with a discernible shape, sufficient to allow us some shared language and public behavior. We no longer have that, either collectively or even in most of our ethnic and religious subgroups. It is a great loss. Every great culture has had a characteristic view of death, ordinarily accompanied by public rituals, customary practices, and time-honored patterns of communal grief. This understanding has provided those cultures with ways of interpreting death, consoling and supporting their members who are encountering it, and giving it a solid and public place in their people's everyday lives. Above all, they have related the question of death to other important categories of life, blending them into a more or less coherent whole. The most important among such categories, I believe, are the self, nature, society, and medicine.

The relationship of death to the self, to the way we think about our individual fate, is the most central issue. Who am I that I must one day die? That question provokes still others, for the way we move toward our death, ordinarily through the door of illness, will force us to confront the problem of suffering, of the evil that sickness, pain, fear, and despair can bring into our lives. What are we to make of them? Nothing less than the meaning of our mortality—the tension between our desire to live and the knowledge that we must get sick and die—is at stake.

Yet if the self must be at the center of our concerns—I must die as well as you—that self is set within a body, and that body within and as a part of nature. What is our relationship to nature, which brings life and death to all organic creatures, but is nevertheless remarkably malleable to human inventiveness? Are we nature's slave or its master? Should it be our guide to the living of a life and the dying of a death, or can we make of them what we will? Can death be shaped to our own ends, its sovereign power domesticated?

Just as we are embodied individual selves, we are also social selves. We live in a society, and, however unique our individuality, social values will shape us and provide us as well with a context of symbols and possibilities for working out our personal destinies. How my society thinks about death, and articulates its perception in its rituals and practices, will shape the way it responds to my dying, and the way it supports me and gives public voice to my struggle with mortality. I will in turn take my own understanding of death in part from that social tutoring.

The relationship of death to the self, to nature, and to society are ancient issues, but once again in need of a fresh look because of one additional, more recent, consideration. Modern medicine, a creature of the eighteenth-century Enlightenment brought to maturity in the second half of the twentieth century, now has remarkable power to change the conditions of our dying and the illnesses that precede it. Yet that power changes everything else as well. It seems to open up radically new possibilities in thinking about who we are, and about the natural and social worlds in which we exist. Those worlds can never quite be the same again, forever altered by scientific visions of change and transformation. The place, then, of medical science in shaping the way we think about death must be added to any serious effort to shape a new cultural understanding of death, a wild card of not yet fully understood influence.

Something else has also come to grip my feeling and imagination. Central to the recent struggles over the care of the dying, and the euthanasia debate, has been the powerful value of personal control over one's life and death. Like scientific medicine, this is a characteristically modern idea, born in part of the desire to throw over the tyranny of repressive ideologies and governments, which presume to own our lives and tell us how we should live. This idea is no less generated by the belief that it is good and proper for us to control our own bodies and to take arms against a repressive, sometimes destructive, nature.

This quest for personal control has been present for many decades, but of late it has taken on an almost driven quality. Nothing seems so feared as the loss of self-determination. It is probably the most dominant issue in the public debate about appropriate laws and policies on the care of the critically ill and dying, taking its rise from the powerful trend over the last century to give patients a choice about their medical treatment and the termination of that treatment; that trend is itself part of a larger drive for more control in all parts of our lives. The passion for control is vividly present in the fears, anxieties, and indignation of a public that has become increasingly terrorized at the prospect of a life that will end stripped of dignity, the victim of a raw and cruel nature, or impersonal medical bureaucracies, or nervous doctors, or guilt-ridden families, or all of them together.

However understandable, I have come to think that the preoccupation with control has become both subtly demeaning and socially troubling. I want to try to show why in this book, but I do so in the face of some imposing obstacles. One of those obstacles is my own temperament, characteristically modern. I am not inclined to let life roll over me, drifting with the flow of things. No. I like to manage my life carefully, to live by schedules, to get my work done on time, and to anticipate and pre-emptively neutralize surprises and interruptions.

Yet I am troubled about those traits, however much I have embraced them. I have grown to admire much more than I did in the past those who live in a different way, who are prepared to give to me the kind of time I would never, my eye on my watch, readily give to them. They have come to seem to me more supple, wiser, better able to live with themselves and others, and to live with the bodies that nature gave them. Most important, people like that seem to me better able to face the threat of death and to cope with it when the time comes. They seem not to feel that losing control over their bodies and fates is the worst thing that can happen to them. They seem even more to fear becoming the kind of persons who would think such a loss of control the worst thing that could happen to them. I have come to admire that.

Even so, I am hardly prepared to relinquish all control, which has its own virtues and congenialities. What is the best balance between control and relinquishment, and what is the difference between a reasonable concern with control and a sickly preoccupation with it? I have been trying to answer these questions about my own life, and about how I should begin approaching my own death. I would hope to engage others in the same worry even if they arrive at a different conclusion from the one I am proposing.

Another obstacle of consequence is that, whether we want to or not, modern medicine increasingly forces us to make choices, to take some charge of our medical care. Should I or should I not have the operation my doctor advises? Should I or should I not chance taking a drug that may help me but at the price of some unpleasant side-effects? Should I or should I not want to go on a respirator to relieve my breathing problems when my doctor is not quite sure whether she can ever wean me off of it? Should I or should I not spend our family savings to seek out a costly, experimental cancer treatment, which may or may not work? To have a choice is to have some control, even a choice to do nothing. We cannot avoid controlling our lives to some extent, even if we would prefer passivity.

In trying to consider these matters, I gradually became conscious of what I take to be a basic, far-reaching division of thought about death that marks our era. Is death to be understood as within, or outside of, human life? It is said, often enough, that death is a "part of life." But what does that phrase, almost a cliché, mean? It has been explored much less than it should be. That exploration inexorably leads to perhaps the most troubling problem of all—how we are to find meaning in death, if there is any meaning to be found.

Even if we can make some sense of the larger questions of control, death, and meaning, we will be left with difficult problems in the way we live our lives. They are intimate and unavoidable. How and when should I want to die? How much pain and suffering should I be willing to bear, and for what reason? What do I owe others in my dying, especially those who would still have me with them if they could? When I am in doubt about my living or dying, where should I locate the benefit of doubt, toward life or death? What kind of person should I be to ask questions of that kind? A person who insists on control of death as well as of life? What kind of person would that make me? As I think about my dying, and the private life that forms the shaping background for it, what are my obligations to the larger society? Can I make an unlimited claim on my fellow citizens to pay, through their taxes and insurance premiums, whatever it takes to keep me alive as long as I (not they) have decided I still have good reasons to live? Can I, for that matter, even make an unlimited claim upon my own family? Can I bring them to destitution to keep me alive, or (if money is not at stake) ask them to sacrifice their time and emotional welfare painfully for my sake?

Whatever better understanding we achieve with those questions must then be woven into a fabric whose strands—reflections on the self, nature, society, fate, and medical science—are pleasing to the mind and also provide some warmth against the chill wind of death. We have tried to make do with death in recent years by working to change the law and medical behavior, and to refine our moral thinking in the face of new dilemmas. That is not enough. However valuable and necessary, such an effort must be rooted more solidly. Just that is my goal here.

If such an effort could succeed, some cautious optimism would be in order. Despite many sad and unfortunate cases, my own experience has been that most people already die reasonably decent deaths. Much to my surprise, for I always assumed my experience was an aberration, some recent studies support my observations, at least with elderly persons. For a large majority, the last year of life is tolerable.[2] That is good news, even if none of us can know whether we will be among the unlucky minority whose death is of a kind no one would want. And it is not illusory to think that the percentage who fall into that minority can be reduced.

The plan of this book is as follows. In the first three chapters I attempt to provide an analysis of our present situation—not good—and why we got here. We have been beset with illusions, and I try to identify them. In chapter 1, I examine why the care of the dying, and the termination of treatment, have proved to be such enduringly difficult issues despite intensive reform efforts. In chapter 2, I turn my attention to the kinds of puzzles and pitfalls that some mistaken views of nature, and our relationship as mortal human beings to that nature, have introduced into our collective thinking about death. In chapter 3, I take up the most recent drive for enhanced personal control, the call for a legalization of active euthanasia and assisted suicide.

In the second half of the book, I offer some alternative approaches to the problems earlier identified. They are meant to include the ingredients necessary to devise a more reasonable, coherent, and supportive set of values and culture in which our dying can take place than the one created by our present illusions. In chapter 4, I take on the question of control. What place should a desire for control have in the way we shape a view of the self? In chapter 5, I directly address the problem of meaning, and especially how meaning is to be discovered, or fashioned, out of a common understanding of death as a great human evil. Is it? And if so, what kind of evil? In chapter 6, I examine medical technology and the way in which we might best use that technology to live better with the reality of death. I conclude the book with some further reflections on the meaning of death in our personal and communal lives and the future of medical science, ever working—wittingly or not—to influence that meaning.

This book is not meant to be a policy manual, a treatise on needed legal reforms, or an exercise in moral casuistry. There are many valuable works already available for these purposes.[3] My aim is to rethink some of the foundations of policy and morality, not to work out the details of specific laws. I hope I say enough in chapter 6, however, to indicate how I think such work might in general best proceed. By the same token, my relative lack of attention to some vexing legal problems should not be taken as a sign that I think them unimportant. They are important, but the spur for this book has been my uneasiness about some of the larger issues that have been neglected in the public discussion and yet serve importantly to set up and structure the way we think about death.

In a number of ways, I continue here the search I initiated in two earlier books, that of trying to understand how we should live with our mortality, and how medicine should help us do so. Even though the explicit focus of *Setting Limits: Medical Goals in an Aging Society* (1987) was on the meaning of old age and the allocation of resources to the elderly, it was also about the relationship between aging and mortality. In *What Kind of Life: The Limits of Medical Progress* (1990), the focus was on the allocation of health-care resources for all age groups, and the design of a reasonable, fair health-care system. But running through it was the strong thread of my interest in the relationship of health, mortality, and human happiness. In this book, I turn directly to the personal questions: how may we best understand and live with our mortality, with the fact that we will and must get sick and die? I suspect that this is what I have been leading up to all the time, though I was not at first aware of it.

I have not hesitated to use my own personal experience to bring forth some of my perspectives. This is my life I am trying to talk about, not just the lives of other people. I have not seen all forms of death or the various possible responses to death. I can only hope that, by relating my own experiences from time to time, I will at least provoke some thoughts about how we may best move back and forth between our personal life and mortality and larger questions of social policy. The problem of death cuts deeply, but too often in reading interesting works by others on the matter I have been wondering what, in their hidden non-academic, nonmedical hearts, they really think and feel about it all. I have tried to reveal that about myself here, but I cannot say I have yet come to the bottom of it. I hope I have some years yet to think further about it. I would sooner write about death than experience it.

Chapter 1

THE FIRST ILLUSION:
MASTERING OUR MEDICAL
CHOICES

Sometimes we are lost and know it. The signposts are unfamiliar and point to places unknown. We realize we must stop and find a new way. At other times, we seem to be following the approved map and yet make little progress. Our doubts and hesitations grow. Where are we going? Just this kind of uncertainty is now appropriate for the unending human effort to understand and pacify death. We have as a culture badly lost our way in that effort, but the air is so full of reform plans, so rich with court decisions and regulatory schemes, that it is easy to be misled. We seem to be doing everything right, working to change those laws and medical practices thought to stand in the way of a tolerable death.

Yet there is, barely below the surface, a remarkable and rising degree of anxiety about dying—not necessarily death as such, but the combination of an extended critical illness gradually transformed into an extended dying.[1] That anxiety is in great part based upon the growing difficulty in making a clear determination that a patient is dying, and that nothing more of life-extending benefit can be done. It is exacerbated by a widespread fear that modern medical death can strip a person of choice and dignity. The anxiety is surprisingly unallayed by the rhetorical potency of the confident slogans that fill the air, "death with dignity" at the top of the list. It is as if, despite that talk, we all understand well enough in some attic of our mind that the kind of illness and dying we are likely to face with modern medicine may refuse to be nicely managed and regulated. We are also half aware that we live in a society increasingly scant in those cultural resources necessary to sustain our interior life as we struggle to make sense of our endings. Reform, yes. Consolation and reassurance, not necessarily, and perhaps not at all.

Where are we? In part we are in an ancient and familiar place, one that leads us to ask that oldest of all questions: how are we, in the secrecy and depth of our own lives, to make sense of our decline and death? Three great struggles of the self with mortality await each of us. There is the struggle to deal with the threat of illness and accident, and sooner or later its reality. That threat reminds me that my body is always at risk of sickness or disability, that things can and will go wrong. I also recognize that, as a self, I will age, that in those spots and wrinkles and aches—in that changing face in the mirror—I have already aged, and that I am destined to become, as W. B. Yeats put it, "a tattered coat upon a stick."[2] I know, finally, that I will as a self someday be dead, that I will be no more, that I will disappear from the face of the earth. I no less know that, before this happens, I must cross the fearful border between life and death.

There was a time when those three threats to the self were often distinct and separable. One could die of a sudden, young and healthy until death struck; of course that still happens to some in our society, especially those young males taken by accident or random violence. Yet most of us will now live into old age, so that illness, aging, and death will accompany one another, imperceptibly blending together. Because we are aging, we are at a rising risk of illness, and because of that risk, we face an increased threat and eventual certainty of death. When we think of death now, it cannot, and probably should not, be so distinctly separated from the biological decline that old age brings with it.

That is not everyone's death by any means, but it is one that most of us can likely expect, barring bad luck or misadventure.

In parallel with the self that must live with its prospect of illness, aging, and death is the self that moves back and forth between its own good and needs and those of others. There is the self that reflects upon its own life and destiny, trying to understand things and endure them. It is a self full of narrow interests— "What is good for me?," "What do I want (whether good for me or not)?"—and full of yearnings, asking, "What kind of person am I?," and "What kind of person do I want to become?" This is the self that looks inward. There is also the social self. It gauges its relationship with others, wanting to know how to live with them and what it should hope, or ask, or demand of them. The latter self can focus its moral lens on the small universe of family and friends, or on the larger one of society and the public space. It can ask, "What kind of citizen do I want to be?," and "What kind of society do I wish to see take shape?" In reality, of course, the private and public selves are in constant exchange, even argument. How should I balance my private interests against the claims of others? Narcissism struggles with altruism; the insistent clamor of desires and wants wrestles with the claims of morality.

To these old struggles has been added the force and power of modern medicine. By changing our bodies and their prospects, medicine changes the self and its expectations as well. I know that I am likely to live a longer and healthier life than my grandparents, and when I become sick I will have a better chance of surviving. Medical powers and possibilities have become the constant companion of the self in its effort to live with mortality.

A Tame Death

Yet we have become ambivalent about that companionship, by turns eager and troubled, desperate to have it but fearful that it will get the better of us, bringing us a death of a kind we do not want at a time we do not want, much later than it should have occurred. In response to that ambivalence, without knowing it, without using quite that language, we have come to feel only now the loss of what the late French historian Philippe Ariès called a "tame" death.[3] By that he meant a death that was tolerable and familiar, affirmative of the bonds of community and social solidarity, expected with certainty and accepted without crippling fear. That kind of human ending, common to most people throughout history until recently, Ariès contrasted with the "wild" death of technological medicine. The latter death—which began to occur in the nineteenth century—is marked by undue fear and uncertainty, by the presence of medical powers not quite within our mastery, by a course of decline that may leave us isolated and degraded. It is wild because it is alien from, and outside of, the cycle of life, because modern technology makes its course highly uncertain, and because it seems removed from a full, fitting presence in the life of the community.

What is the "tame death" of which Ariès wrote? "The tame death," he argued, "is the oldest death there is."[4] To make his case, he opens his great history of death in Western culture, *The Hour of Our Death*, with what might strike us as an implausible example of an ordinary death in the Middle Ages, that of the knight Roland, described in the *Chanson de Roland*. Death is known to be coming, is then prepared for, and takes place calmly amid a circle of friends and acquaintances. Yet Roland's death is not an exceptional death, even though he is a knight. It distills popular and oral traditions of a reality—the "unchronicled death throughout the long ages of the most ancient history, and perhaps prehistory."[5] It was a death marked above all by three distinct features. The notion of "familiar simplicity"[6] captures two of them, its public character the third. Death was familiar because, with short life spans making death an event among every age group, it was a steady and routine part of daily life. It was marked by simplicity because of its ritualized, unchanging features over the centuries, little altered by medical or social change.

A passage from Solzhenitsyn's *Cancer Ward* reflects the same idea, one that lingered on well into the nineteenth and early twentieth centuries: "The old folk," his character Yefrem says in describing the way they faced death, "didn't puff themselves up or fight against it and brag that they weren't going to die—they took death *calmly.* They didn't stall squaring things away, they prepared themselves quietly and in good time, deciding who would have the mare, who the foal . . . and they departed easily, as if they were now moving into a new house."[7] A comparable perspective can be found closer to home. It is illustrated by an incident reported from a hospital during the American Civil War. In these institutions, notable for their filth and their poor staffing, and filled with the cries and moans of the maimed and wounded, " 'The patients would see that the doctor gave them up,' a Confederate steward recalled, 'and would ask me about it. I would tell them the truth. I told one man that and he asked 'How long?' I said 'Not over twenty minutes.' He did not show any fear. They never do. He put his hand up so and closed his eyes with his own fingers and he stretched himself out and crossed his arms over his breast. 'Now fix me,' he said. I pinned the toes of his stockings together. That was the way we lay corpses out, and he died in a few minutes. His face looked as pleasant as if he was asleep. And many is the time the boys have fixed themselves that way before they died."[8]

Or consider the words of the seventeenth-century poet Ben Jonson, in "An Elegy on the Lady Jane Paulet":

> *With gladness Temper'd her sad parents tears;*
> *Made her friends joys, to get above their fears.*
> *And, in her last act, taught the standers by,*
> *With admiration and applause, to die!*[9]

A third important feature of the tame death was its public character. "The vile and ugly death of the Middle Ages," Ariès writes, "is . . . the secret death that is without witness or ceremony: the death of the traveler on the road, or the man who drowns in the river, or the stranger whose body is found at the edge of a field, or even the neighbor who is struck down for no reason."[10] A tame death, by contrast, is public and ceremonial. It takes place amid a circle of family, friends, and children, and in many places it was acceptable for strangers to come in off the street to be with the dying person. Only perhaps at the very end, for a few hours only, was a person left alone; otherwise, nothing was more important than to keep the dying fully and richly within the human community until the last moments.

The motive behind the desire for a public death was not simply to comfort the dying, but, more important, to express communal solidarity in the face of death: "It was not only an individual who was disappearing, but society itself that had been wounded and that had to be healed. . . . The rites in the bedroom or those of the oldest liturgy express the conviction that the life of a man is not an individual destiny but a link in an unbroken chain, the biological continuation of a family or a line that begins with Adam and includes the whole human race. . . . Thus, death was not a personal drama but an ordeal for the community. . . . It could not be a solitary adventure but had to be a public phenomenon involving the whole community."[11]

How could a tame death have been possible? Can we, moreover, believe a historical account that sounds just a bit too perfect, too romantic, and makes of death an event too lacking in the fear, the dread, that we have come to associate with it? I have come to think Ariès's account essentially correct. Yet I have been surprised at the resistance many people have to the idea of a tame death in the past, as if it simply could not have been that way. We seem compelled to believe that death *must* have been worse in earlier times, that surely modern medicine must have brought great improvement. Not necessarily.[12] Both biology and history make Ariès's account of a tame death plausible and believable. An important biological fact underlies the picture of death he develops from the historical record. For the most part (as I will develop more on p. 42), people in earlier times typically died of infectious disease of rapid onset and quick crisis; they did in fact die over a relatively short period of time. The long and lingering death of our day was uncommon. This meant that someone could be awake and alert, even if suffering, until the last moments. Death was more a discrete event than a drawn-out, indefinite process. That discreteness made possible— and perfectly plausible in historical retrospect—a public leave- taking, efforts at reconciliation, the disbursing of property, and a formal, final parting with those close to the dying person. Such features were the essence of the ritual.

The biological record makes medically plausible, then, the picture of dying Ariès develops. But it is no less important to note the emphasis he places on one necessary precondition of a tame death. Death is not, and should not become, a glorious event to be sought and embraced. It is an evil. It ruptures the solidarity of the human community. It forces the dying person out of the lives of those around her, a loss both to her and to others. The source of the evil is the "savagery of nature," a nature to be accepted but not romanticized.[13] "Familiarity with death is a form of acceptence of the order of nature."[14] "Death," as Ariès puts it, "may be tamed, divested of the blind violence of natural forces, and ritualized, but it is never experienced as a neutral phenomenon. . . . Resignation was not, therefore, sub- mission to a benevolent nature, or a biological necessity, as it is today, as it was no doubt among the Epicureans or Stoics; rather it is the recognition of an evil inseparable from man."[15]

If modern medicine was itself accepted—its promise was great, its transformation of mortality striking—the wild death it brought was not. That was an unwelcome part of the bargain of medical progress. What was to be done about it? The response has been uncertain and evasive. Ariès's own judgment concern- ing the direction of that response is clear. *The Hour of Our Death* ends on a note of bemused irony: "Medicine reduced pain. . . . The goal glimpsed in the eighteenth century had almost been reached. Evil was no longer part of human nature. . . . It still existed, of course, but outside of man, in certain marginal spaces that morality and politics had not yet colonized, in certain de- viant behaviors such as war, crime, and nonconformity . . . but which one day would be eliminated. . . . But if there is no more evil, what do we do about death? To this question modern society offers two answers. The first is a massive admission of defeat. We ignore the existence of a scandal that we have been unable to prevent; we act as if it did not exist. . . . [The second] is to reduce death to a feigned indifference. Either way, the result is the same: Neither the individual nor the community is strong enough to recognize the existence of death."[16]

Ariès was by no means the only author to strike the note of "the denial of death," the title of Ernest Becker's Pulitzer Prize–winning book of 1973, and anticipated earlier in Geoffrey Gorer's celebrated 1955 article "The Pornography of Death."[17] Gorer first called attention to the peculiar way in which Victorian sexual constraints were gradually overthrown, but those same constraints were used to suppress the public expression of death. To this Becker added an acute analysis of the stratagems used culturally and by the individual unconscious to drive death from our conscious life, simply to declare (without winning) a psychological victory over our fear of dying. He tellingly cites a striking passage written by William James many years earlier: "Let sanguine healthy-mindedness do its best with its strange power of living in the moment and ignoring and forgetting, still the evil background is really there to be thought of, and the skull will grin in at the banquet."[18] Has it always been that way? Not necessarily. The contribution of Philippe Ariès was to show, in the broad historical panorama of Western responses to death, how radical, how truly new, that suppression was. A wild death is not only a technological death, but a hidden, dirty death, one that is shunned, feared, and denied.

The Tame Death Lost

The tame death did not survive. The combination of cultural and religious changes, and the rise of scientific medicine, brought it to an end. By the eighteenth century, life expectancies had begun their shift toward modern standards; they were accelerating still more rapidly by the end of the nineteenth century. The great cultural changes that took place during these centuries showed a move away from the idea of death as a fixed, collective destiny, to one that focused on the death of the isolated self, and from there to the death of the other, the loved one taken away amid grief and with a sense of enduring loss.

Death soon ceased to be simple and familiar. The emergence of nineteenth-century rituals of dramatic mourning, of death pictured as the brutal snatching of the loved one from the unwilling grasp of family and friends, in one way carried on the tradition of death as a communal evil, destroying the fabric of human relationships. But in another way it also signaled a gradual shift to death as a more segregated personal and psychological event, first from the community at large to the family, and then, by the late twentieth century, taken out of the hands of families and put into those of doctors and medical institutions.

The first steps of this transformation were subtle. By the nineteenth century, as so beautifully caught in Tolstoy's story "The Death of Ivan Ilyich," what Ariès calls the "beginning of the lie" appears, the hiding of imminent death from the dying person, the pretense that recovery was just around the corner. "The worst torment," Tolstoy writes of Ivan, "was the lie, this lie that for some reason was accepted by everyone, that he was only sick and not dying, and that if he would only remain calm and take care of himself, everything would be fine. . . . He suffered because they lied and forced him to take part in this deception . . . this lie that degraded the formidable and solemn act of his death."[19] From the beginning of the lie to the individual it was not a long step to the beginning of the lie to the larger society. The rise of the funeral industry, the removal of the body from the home and the adornment of it with the cosmetic veneer of life for ceremonial display, the gradual transformation of grief from a public to a private event, and the elimination of mourning clothes were all ways of hiding death. The emergence of the institutional death in hospitals and nursing homes by the mid-twentieth century was simply one more, albeit highly decisive, way of putting death out of sight.

Why could death no longer be looked straight in the face? Why was it increasingly seen as soiled and indecent, first to be concealed from the dying person and then, parallel with his exclusion from the truth, to be banished altogether from the public space? The most plausible explanation is the transformation of the idea of death in the hands of modern medicine. As early as Francis Bacon, who first called for medicine to seek the cure of disease, and the French *philosophes*, who fostered the scientific ideal of the near-elimination of death altogether, the notion of death as fixed human destiny was dismantled. "The area of the invisible death," Ariès wrote, "is also the area of the greatest belief in the power of technology and its ability to transform man and nature. Our modern model of death was born and developed in places that gave birth to two beliefs: first, the belief in a nature that seemed to eliminate death; next, the belief in a technology that would replace nature and eliminate death the more surely."[20]

Ariès overstates the matter. I doubt that many serious medical researchers have believed that death could be overcome. The deeper belief is of a more subtle kind: that medicine can, in its conquest of disease, remove the unpleasant, distressing *causes* of death, thus transmuting it from a condition to be feared to one that can be managed and tolerated. If death can be socially hidden, and medicine can remove its sting, then it can cease to be of consequence in the lives of individuals or society. This is, ironically, a nascent idea of a tame death, but now not one tamed by acceptance of death as it has been historically—out of control, choosing its own time and place—but of death remodeled, domesticated, and camouflaged by medical technology.

That way has been tried now for at least three or four decades. It is not working. Death has not been pleasingly remodeled or successfully domesticated. That is not the way death has turned out, not at all. Nor is there any good evidence that we will soon see such a nicely polished death. Death is still feared, perhaps more than ever when associated with the chronic, slow-killing diseases of modern mortality, and the fear now more intensely encompasses the course and trajectory of dying. Instead of gaining relief, we have suffered a dual loss.

There is, first, the loss of the familiarity and simplicity that marked the earlier tame death, a death that could be understood as evil yet accepted with a certain resignation and tranquillity—and a death that, in an era of infectious disease, came rapidly and decisively. Though it is handily absent, there is often little simplicity about death today, which is for the most part institutional and requiring a specific decision to discontinue medical treatment (sometimes called a "managed death"). This is the death that increasingly terrorizes us, even as the possibility of management is meant to reassure us. Its uncertainty, its contrived quality, is itself enough to inspire fear and dread.

There is, second, another, no less fearsome, loss. Just as the fatalism, the resigned acceptance of destiny, was dismantled in favor of the medical management of death, so also were all those attendant rituals, habits, and practices that were able to give cultural and religious meaning to death, to give it a familiar place in public and private life. We too easily forget the great value of ritual (and I do not mean just religious ritual): that is, the comfort of knowing how to behave publicly in the presence of death—what to say, how to compose one's face, to whom to speak, and when to speak. When one of our children died as an infant, there was nothing more strained and awkward for my wife and me than trying to respond to those who did not know what to do, those who wanted to say something but had no vocabulary to speak of death, who wanted to give comfort but could do so in no forthright, strong way. More often than not, it was my wife and I who had to help them, to put them at ease as they struggled without success to find a way to talk with us. There was no common resource they could bring to bear to express their grief. There can be nothing worse than concocted, self-conscious ritual, creating a make-believe world of sweetness and light to cover over the harshness of death. But serious customs and rituals, refined over time, can give a shape and context to grief and our understanding of death.

By the time Philippe Ariès had come to the end of his own life, he had seen the effort of the 1960s and 1970s to bring death back on the public stage, to overcome its invisibility, its pornography, as Gorer had described it. He was not greatly impressed. For most people, it still remained hidden, evaded; that was the way our life was organized. For a small elite, it was faced and talked about, but now in terms just a bit too cool, too detached, to ring quite true: "They propose to reconcile death with happiness."[21] Yet the terror has not abated; it has grown. "This should not surprise us," Ariès notes. "Belief in evil was necessary to the taming of death; the disappearance of the belief has restored death to its savage state."[22]

If Philippe Ariès were alive today, he would not find much reason for a revised judgment about the denial of death, nor would he find any serious effort to deal with the questions he left with us. He would, to be sure, observe a great deal of legislative and court activity and an endless amount of talk about dying in the medical journals, the popular media, and the streets. Over the past decade, there have been greatly intensified efforts to establish our right to be allowed to die, and to explore the moral duty we owe to the choice that autonomous moral agents, as we are sometimes called, can make about our dying.

Much of this activity is beneficial, but not enough so. It is surely not what Becker, Ariès, Gorer, and others had in mind when they tried to provoke a renewed consideration of death. Correctly and with profundity, they said that death itself is the issue. That is what we must confront and think about. That is the power of two questions that Ariès left with us, which he himself did not explore. "Is there," he asked, "a permanent relationship between one's idea of death and one's idea of oneself?"[23] His other question was this: "Must we take for granted that it is impossible for our technological culture ever to regain the naive confidence in Destiny which had for so long been shown by simple men when dying?"[24]

The Poverty of Choice

Instead of pursuing questions of that kind, we have discovered
in the language of choice and rights still another kind of evasion,
congenial enough in a society that has an increasingly difficult
time distingushing between the demands of self-understanding
and the demands of civil liberties. Faced with the possibility of
going in different directions with death in the 1960s and 1970s,
we collectively chose to add still another barrier between ourselves and a steady look at death: we chose "choice" about death,
rather than death itself, as the new, supposedly liberating focus.
This was, at the time, a perfectly reasonable response. Many
people were in fact being denied a right to have treatment ter-
minated, and a corrective was needed. It also served most effectively to stimulate public interest and discussion.

Death was, in a sense, taken out of the closet. But instead of
being put forward for common thought and probing, it was put
into the courtroom, turned into a matter of grand human rights.
That is not altogether inappropriate, but is it enough? Can it
even be fully meaningful if it fails to engage the older and deeper
questions about the human significance of death?

Consider in this respect what we have come to. You ask:
"What does death mean?" The answer: "That is for you to
choose." You ask again, not entirely satisfied: "But what should
I think about?" The answer: "That is your right to decide." You
ask once more, by now becoming restless: "What kind of a person
should I be to ask such questions and have such rights?" The
answer: "Who knows?" The more publicly sanctioned our right
to choose death, so it seems, the more buried, the more hidden,
the meaning of that death in our lives, and the more excluded
from any common, public discourse. The more public becomes
the espousal of choice, the more private the content and substance of that choice.

Socially and legally, instead of attempting to stimulate our collective understanding of death, the decisive emphasis has fallen
on establishing a set of rights about our dying that will give us

sovereignty over our bodies. The aim, of course, has been the empowerment of patients to say no to unwanted treatment, to specify conditions for their dying, and to chart by written or oral statements the course of their medical therapies. The *expressed* goal of these efforts, admirable and necessary, has been to remove medical and legal obstacles, then to allow us to shape a death of our own, with our own meaning. Yet there is an ever-present hazard in a culture that too easily mistakes the limited purpose of law for the broader and deeper demands of morality. It is that the aim of overcoming obstacles to choice to make way for meaning will be taken as the end of the matter, the latter task forgotten and slighted, culturally starved of the means of sustenance.

However welcome the legal developments as a way of coping with medicine—and it is *imperative* that they go forward—we must understand that they conduce, even if unwittingly, to misdirecting our gaze and attention. Instead of discussing openly how to think about death and what we might appropriately choose in our dying—a painful and difficult subject—we too frequently and too easily transform the issue into the more distanced, comfortable language of rights and choices: not *how* or *what* we ought to choose, but that we have a right to choose. Even though the supposed aim of choice is to open the way for us to devise and act upon our own meanings, a right to choice that is not complemented and undergirded by rich cultural and moral resources, and incentives to exercise that right wisely, can be vacuous. It can then be just one more way of evading thought about death and, in the process, adding a new terror, that of the need to make a choice in the absence of any signposts for doing so.

There is, in fact, a kind of inverse correlation between the language of meaning and moral substance—the content of choice—and an emphasis on the right to make a choice. As death has been drained of social meaning, the right to control the conditions of dying has been all the more strongly asserted. The demand for control, the unwillingness to accept death as it might present itself if untouched, is not only strong, it has become a passion for many. The only evil greater than one's personal death is increasingly taken to be the loss of control of that death.

Illusions of Mastery

I want to argue, however, that two massive illusions now mark the change I have just described. One of them is the naïve belief that the watchful self, aided by the right laws and medical practices, can master the body by means of carefully controlled medical technology. That self can, it is believed, understand technology well enough to know when and how in the course of dying to find medically the just-right moment to halt it, to say, "No more, stop." The other illusion complements the first: that we can know ourselves and our own wishes well enough to manage ourselves with the same precision with which we would control the technology, that we will understand ourselves well enough to know when to give up the struggle to stay alive. It is as if we can come to know ourselves and our inner world with the same clarity, and the same mastery, that technology gives us over the outer world.

Yet even if we could manage our inner selves better, for which there is no good evidence, the necessity of managing both the self and technology at the same time has turned out to be far harder than anticipated. Consider the recent history of efforts to improve the management of dying and the termination of treatment. The general problem was quickly identified well over two decades ago: since medical technology can prolong lives beyond the point of all sense and value, what can be done to avoid such a result? The response was quick in coming. Stimulated by widespread complaints, by the work of Elisabeth Kübler-Ross, and by numerous ethical and legal committees, the "death-with-dignity" movement was born in the early 1970s. That phrase articulated the conviction that patients have a right to reject life-extending medical care if they so desire, and it expressed the hope that medical care at the end of life could focus on the patient as a person, not merely as a collection of failing organs. A now familiar three-part reform agenda accompanied that broad goal.

The first part was to give patients a greater power of self-determination, and specifically to do so by means of advance directives, most commonly the ("living will" or durable-power-of-attorney legislation.[25] Under the former, patients can specify in a written statement precisely what forms of medical treatment they do, or do not, want during their terminal illness. Under the latter, which is more favored in recent years, they can designate someone to act in their behalf. Both are triggered by loss of patient decisionmaking capacity. All of the states now have advance-directive legislation.[26]

The second part of the reform agenda was to institute "hospice" programs throughout the country. Patterned on the original work of Cicely Saunders in Great Britain, their idea has been to provide comfort and palliation for the dying, not aggressive medical treatment. Only specially developed facilities or specialized home-care programs, and well-trained people, can provide this kind of alternative to the typical medical institution. The hospice idea caught on and, by the middle of the 1980s, qualified for support under the federal Medicare program.[27]

The third part of the reform effort related to an idea at the heart of the hospice movement: that special efforts and training are necessary to help doctors and other health-care workers focus on the patient as an individual, to learn how to curb the appetite for technological dominance when it is inappropriate, and how to accept death. Dozens of medical schools now incorporate some efforts to provide such an education.[28]

What has been the effect of these three reforms? The most obvious answer is: much, much less than everyone had hoped. But that response is too general. A more careful answer has to be given at two levels, looking at the actual effects of the reforms on medical practice, and their more general effects in allaying public anxiety. Their effect on medical practice has been, at best, modest, and surely so in comparison with the early high expectations. They have made, and can increasingly make, important contributions to many individuals, but they are unlikely to more generally transform the way most of us will die.

Advance directives have been signed by less than 15 percent of the American public, despite widespread publicity and discussion. Numerous and intense efforts to increase that number significantly have not been notably successful; it remains a phenomenon mainly of the affluent, well-educated middle class, and it is by no means anywhere near universal even among them. Numerous problems of interpretation and implementation have appeared over the years, further limiting their impact.[29]

The hospice movement had an early period of vigorous growth but for some time now has seen a relatively slow growth pattern. In 1992, there were some 1,874 hospice programs, with one hundred added since 1991. They served over two hundred thousand patients in 1992.[30] Recognition soon came, moreover, that it was of greatest value to those suffering from cancer, a disease whose downward course could be better foreseen and managed by hospice than, say, heart disease or Alzheimer's disease.

As for the practice of physicians at the bedside, progress has been hard to measure. If there has been improvement in the attitudes and practices of physicians toward the dying, and there has, it has by no means been so striking as to be decisively transforming. Doctors still do not, as a rule, talk comfortably and directly with patients about death. They are still, in general, not inclined to initiate discussions with patients on the subject. A worry about malpractice, a zest for technology, a deep-seated moral belief in the need to prolong life, and the pressure of families and others still often lead to overtreatment and an excessive reliance on technology.

Have public anxieties abated in the wake of twenty years of legal, social, and medical reform efforts? Has it become easier to stop treatment? The answer to both questions is, I believe, no. The rapid shift of public opinion on assisted suicide and active euthanasia provides one piece of indirect evidence for that judgment.[31] There is little public confidence that the critically ill will be able to withstand the force of advanced medicine, or that they will have much control over their dying. A more direct correlation is not easy to prove, but there is much suggestive evidence. Just about everyone can tell plentiful stories these days about friends or family members treated excessively or pointlessly. They could not understand why the treatment was pressed forward. It is not always easy even for physicians themselves to explain. Many physicians do know the wishes of their patients. They do not want to do for their patients more than what is desired or useful. Yet many physicians nonetheless tell me that they find decisions to stop treatment harder now than they were twenty years ago, both morally and technically.

Many patients and their families, lulled by the possession of an advance directive, find to their dismay that it does not do them as much good as they expected.[32] Sometimes doctors just ignore such directives. More often, and more significantly, the nature of the terminal illness makes it exceedingly hard to know when to invoke the provisions of the directive. As one friend tearfully told me, her mother has been suffering for years from congestive heart failure; though advance directives were in hand, they were useless to the patient and everyone around her. The doctors have simply not been able to determine, in crisis after crisis, whether she is dying. Given that uncertainty, the provisions of the advance directive could not be invoked. Time and again, I have been told similar stories, and this impression has been strengthened by anecdotes and other information provided me by various audiences and groups to whom I have spoken in the last couple of years.

Technological Brinkmanship

At the center of these difficulties in reform is an intensification, over the same period, of what I will call technological brinkmanship. By that I mean there has been a powerful clinical drive to push technology as far as possible to save life while, at the same time, preserving a decent quality of life. It is well recognized by now that, if medical technology is pushed too far, a person can be harmed, that there is a line that should not be crossed. I define "brinkmanship" as the gambling effort to go *as close to that line as possible* before the cessation or abatement of treatment. Common sense seems to dictate such a course: aggressively work to prolong life until it becomes futile, or harmful, to continue doing so; then, just as boldly, halt life-extending treatment. But this seemingly obvious strategy assumes an ability to manage technology and its consequences with a delicacy and precision that medicine simply does not possess and may never possess. The effort to go as close to the line as possible is itself the problem, resting on naïve illusions and false assumptions.

Note that the problem I am pointing to here is not the abuse of technology, or the thoughtless and insensitive use of technology to extend life beyond all point or reason. I am instead identifying the main problem as the belief that we can manage our technology and its effects with the precision necessary to make brinkmanship succeed. That strategy has not worked well and, as presently conceived, cannot work well. The result of this continuing failure is the violence of death by technological attenuation, a stretching to the limit and beyond the power of technology to extend the life of organ systems independent of the welfare of the persons to whom they belong. That violence is occasioned by otherwise well-intentioned efforts to use technology to combat death. The brinkmanship itself is dangerous, not simply the failures that can result when it is not successful; the brinkmanship itself increases dramatically the likelihood of failure. That brinkmanship, moreover, is a source of the frequently reported impersonality of hospital deaths. Because of the focus on technological intervention, the human relationships are often neglected, judged less important, more dispensable, than the necessity of high-quality technical work. Machines and lab results and scanners become the center of attention; they replace conversation with the patient.

In particular, brinkmanship fails to reckon with two potent

realities, each of which conspires to make it hard to locate the point at which the brinkmanship should stop, and just as hard to work up the will to stop once this point has been identified. The two realities are the vanishing line between life and death, which makes it difficult to determine when to stop the use of technology, and the continuing profound public and medical ambivalence about what is wanted and valued in coping with illness and dying. The combination of these two realities creates a powerful resistance to efforts to struggle against the violence of a death by technological attenuation. They work together, reinforcing each other.

The Vanishing Line Between Life and Death

The signal characteristic of most illnesses in the past was their rapidity of onset and speed of resolution. The pattern of illness and fatality between 1600 and 1870 was in striking contrast to that in our own times. The main causes of death were dysentery, cholera, influenza, plague, smallpox, typhoid fever, and tuberculosis.[33] If one did not die of those diseases, one got well. Sickness was a relatively temporary phenomenon, not chronic. With bacillary dysentery, if death was to be the outcome, it would come within two to four days; the entire course of the disease was only one week. With cholera, death could come within a few hours, and one week was a typical course for that illness as well. In the case of typhoid fever, it could be a few days or up to two weeks. With the plague, the disease could last longer than four weeks, but death was most likely in the first and third weeks.[34] To be sure, some indolent illnesses occurred (especially TB), and some of the slower diseases of old age (e.g., cancer), but the ordinary fatal illness would rarely last longer than eight weeks.[35]

We might naturally assume that, because death was more frequent, more indiscriminate in the age of its victims, sickness and lingering illness were more common. That was not true: they are far more common today. Since most earlier illnesses and deaths were caused by infectious disease, accident, or injury, they were faster and more intensive in their course, and more rapid in their lethal outcome. If a person recovered, by contrast, that recovery was likely to be both speedier and less likely to produce lingering harms or disabilities. In the absence of effective medical treatment, it was left to the body to do its own unaided recovery. If it could do so, it did so rapidly. If it could not, death would come quickly.

The conquest of infectious disease, and the emergence of effective therapies, together brought a striking change. Beginning about 1870, life expectancy rapidly increased, stimulated in great part by a drop in infant- and child-mortality rates. But as the average length of a life increased, so did the amount of sickness. A longer life came to mean a life marked by a greater incidence of illness, and a greater length of illness once incurred: the price of a longer life has been a sicker life.[36] Death now principally comes from the chronic and degenerative diseases of aging. Sudden death, when it occurs, is most likely going to result from accidents or criminal violence.

Although people can and do of course still die of sudden heart attacks or strokes, or rapidly spreading cancer, the chronic diseases are more characteristically slow to develop (the cumulative insults resulting in cancer or heart disease may take years) and slow to kill. The average length of time from the detected onset of a fatal cancer and the resultant death is estimated to be three years; in Alzheimer's disease it is about seven years. Some heart conditions last for years before claiming their victims. Diabetes may eventually kill, but slowly, by gradually ruining the circulatory system or destroying the kidneys. Beyond the slowness of their natural course, medical interventions can of course strikingly prolong the disease and offset the likely fatal outcome: insulin for diabetes, dialysis for victims of end-stage renal disease, heart drugs and surgery for heart disease, and drugs and surgery for cancer. When natural organs fail, artificial organs or devices can increasingly be brought to bear. The most striking result of the success of medical technology is the very strong trend toward the combination of longer lives and worsening health. Despite efforts to reduce the burden of sickness, sickness has increased as life has lengthened, and both the duration of illness and the number of disabilities have increased as well.

When, in this process, is a patient dying? That becomes harder and harder to say. Predictions of death, unless virtually imminent, become increasingly problematic. Who among us does not know of someone, stricken by a supposedly fatal cancer or heart disease, who is still alive and active months or years after a predicted death? The slow, but variable, course of most chronic diseases alone makes it difficult to say when death is on its way. When to that uncertainty is added the further impact of life-extending therapy, whose purpose is to stretch the borderline and the practice of brinkmanship, whose purpose is to resist the idea of a fixed limit, the location of the gate between life and death becomes more indeterminate.

I conclude that it is becoming increasingly useless to base decisions concerning whether to terminate treatment on some medical determination that a patient "is dying." To determine well in advance that an illness is "terminal" has always been difficult, and is increasingly so today. But it is also growing harder to say that death is "imminent," meaning within a few hours or days. Many hospital rules and policy statements make use of the distinction between patients whose death is imminent and those whose death is not. The late theologian Paul Ramsey spoke of persons "seized by their own dying" to capture the distinction, and another common, popular formulation has distinguished between "extending life" and "extending death."[37] But medical progress is rendering all of these distinctions problematic, of less and less use for actual decisionmaking. My own informal survey has found, in fact, that the principal reason for the failure of advance directives to allow for decisions as good as hoped for has been medical uncertainty about when to invoke them, much more than unwillingness on the part of physicians to honor them. The reason for this uncertainty, which I believe is growing, is twofold. First, judgments about whether patients are "dying" are always probabilistic in nature—i.e., based on estimates of the probable odds of death's coming; technological developments increasingly obscure the clear determination of those odds. New, improved therapeutics will make it harder to predict that a disease will inevitably be fatal, and whether—even if inevitably fatal—death can be delayed to some significant extent. Second, the uncertain nature of the odds tends to play into the hands of a clinical nervousness that makes termination decisions difficult and threatening. A physician can, reasonably, say that he is not certain a patient is "dying"—until more efforts to save the patient have been made, and still more again.

A primary difficulty can be described as follows. Even if there is less, say, than a 5-to-10-percent chance that a particular treat- ment will save the life of a critically ill patient, there will often be no clear way to determine which patient will be among that 5 to 10 percent. In order to spare them an unnecessary death, it will be necessary to treat all patients *as if* they may be among the minority that will be benefited.[38] I am not denying that there can and will be some reasonably clear cases. I am only contending that, with medical advances, they are and will continue to be fewer and fewer. Physiological "dying" as a moral standard for terminating treatment will, therefore, become less and less useful. It may be possible still to use it when death is only a few days off. But, increasingly, the important treatment decisions will need to come well before this point; and that is just where the uncertainty continues to grow.

If a determination of "dying" will be increasingly difficult to make, are there any alternative standards that might be used? They will have to be multiple and complex in the future, a combination of quality-of-life judgments based on potential pa- tient welfare, and standards devised to terminate treatment be- fore the process of dying is itself deformed by technological attenuation. Most critically, a different stance will be necessary about where to locate the burden of doubt, in favor of or against continued treatment. I propose some standards in chapters 5 and

6. The old question was: when is a patient dying, and thus a candidate for the abatement of lifesaving treatment? The new question should be: at what point, or within what range, should lifesaving treatment be abated to enhance the likelihood of a good death?

Nor is the difficulty of determining when someone is "dying" the end of the matter. In earlier deaths from infectious disease, the body and the mind would more or less succumb at the same time. A person's life might end with a coma, or delirium, but that would be for a relatively short time only: pneumonia, or urinary-tract infection, or gangrene would bring an end to the body. Not so any longer. The mind can be long gone, either in advanced dementia, where there still remains a simulacrum of language, feeling, and cognition, or in a persistent vegetative state, where all consciousness is lost, the higher brain destroyed. Whether through relatively simple antibiotics to control infections of a once-lethal kind, or through the elaborate apparatus of artificial respiration or nutrition, the body can be maintained, the relatively intact home of a mind and consciousness long demolished.

Just as the line between the life and the death of the body can be attenuated, stretched to a point of invisibility, so also can the relationship of the mind and the body. In the absence of definitive tests for electrical activity in the higher brain, the cerebral cortex, at no point can it be definitively said when the mind, and thus the person, exists no more. It happens, we suppose, but we do not know when.

What technological advances have done, then, is to change the nature of illness to increase the degree and duration of sickness once contracted, to render near-invisible the line between extending a life and extending a death, and then—as a final touch—to render invisible the borderline between a living person and a biologically functioning body. As Philippe Ariès could say almost two decades ago: "Death has been dissected, cut to bits by a series of little steps, which finally make it impossible to know which step was the real death, the one in which consciousness was lost, or the one in which breathing stopped. All these little silent deaths have replaced the great dramatic act of death, and no one any longer has the strength or patience to wait over a period of weeks for a moment which has lost a part of its meaning."[39]

The various changes together can be summed up as follows:

- longer lives and worse health
- longer illnesses and slower deaths
- longer aging and increased dementia

These changes have forced a new definition of death, from cessation of heart and lung activity to whole-brain death. They have also brought closer to hand a still more refined criterion in the death of the cerebral cortex and have led to enormous definitional (not to mention moral) problems about the nature and timing of death. These changes have also made far more complex other conceptual and definitional issues, important for both policy and personal purposes. When is further treatment "useless"? What is medical "futility"? Hardly anyone disagrees with the seemingly simple and noncontroversial notion that medical treatment should cease when it becomes futile. Yet what should be the standard for measuring futility? That the treatment will no longer benefit the body? But it may, nonetheless, be desired by the patient and keep alive the patient's hope. It is not, in that sense, futile at all; it may bring a benefit to the patient as a person. Is treatment futile because the odds against its working are low? Still, for a patient it may seem well worth the gamble. The uncertain outcome of some established therapies, which may work now and then in seemingly hopeless cases, or of experimental therapies, whose outcomes are not known, can render the notion of "futility" a wraith, coming in and out of the mist of certainty and probability. Technological advances constantly change the probabilities of therapeutic outcome. Even if agreement can be reached on patient welfare, medical advances can continually shift the bodily component of that idea. Technological brinkmanship rests on a belief in what turns out to be a more and more elusive capacity to match technological possibility carefully with bodily reality; and technology itself has brought that about.

"Why is it now so hard to die a tame death?" we might well ask. Here is now a first reason: because medicine finds it harder and harder to locate the line between living and dying, and thus to know when to stop treatment. Improved advance directives will not necessarily improve that situation.

Words and Deeds, Wishes and Actions

One popular and apparently persuasive belief has gained considerable ground in recent years. Most people, but particularly the elderly, it is said, do not want aggressive lifesaving efforts made when they are dying. They want comfort and palliation only. There are many reasons, however, to be doubtful about the precise meaning and import of such statements, much less to treat them as wholly reliable indicators of what people will actually choose when they are critically ill. At best, they may be reasonably reliable general guides to certain negative outcomes that are not wanted—for instance, great pain or extended coma—but be less reliable about the choices people will make under more ambiguous circumstances. General statements about what people *say* they do not want must be contrasted with other data that indicate that, when a critical illness is at hand, people most often do want many forms of aggressive medical treatment. There are two issues to be sorted out here. The first is whether what people say they want in advance of a terminal illness is a good predictor of what they will want when it actually occurs. The second is what people actually *mean* when they make statements about the kind of medical care they want or do not want.

My thesis is as follows. Futile medical treatment is indeed ordinarily not wanted, but useful treatment *is* wanted. That would seem obvious enough, except that "useful" treatment is interpreted in such a broad fashion that it is often wanted even when its utility is highly marginal, and when the quality of life it provides is slight to vanishing. For practical purposes, it is this desire for useful treatment, however slight in value, that is most important, *not* the declared rejection of futile treatment. The consequences of the difference are important. Given the growing effectiveness of medical therapies at the margin of life and death, and the increased difficulty of pinpointing the line between living and dying, medical and lay ambivalence and uncertainty are necessarily intensified. One result is that people can say one thing when well, but behave in an apparently different way when sick. If careful attention is paid, however, to what they are really saying when well, there may be less of a contradiction than might otherwise seem true. But it also means that there should be considerably less confidence than is commonly expressed that simply giving people a choice about terminating treatment will actually result in a dramatic change in treatment patterns. That is less likely.

What do people say they want? A composite picture developed from public-opinion surveys show that they overwhelmingly would want life-support systems withheld or withdrawn if there is no hope of recovery or if there is great pain.[40] One could easily gather, from that data, that most people, and particularly the elderly, are highly resistant to aggressive high-technology, life-extending treatment. But the survey results on general attitudes toward treatment must be compared with some other evidence, and some other survey results. There is a considerable body of data to show that, in recent years, the elderly have in fact accepted a sharp increase in high-technology care. The fastest-growing group making use of kidney dialysis is the elderly, and that use grows even though there is often a poor outcome. "Older and sicker" is the general trend. Parallel evidence exists for an increase in the use of open-heart and bypass surgery, and there has been a gradual increase in the age of organ-transplantation recipients as well.[41]

Another kind of evidence pertinent here is the studies that ask, not general questions, but whether patients would want specific kinds of treatments. Most striking are those surveys showing a surprising willingness on the part of patients who previously endured an ICU episode to undergo still another round to save their lives. The overwhelming majority would be willing to undergo such treatment again—even to achieve a very slight prolongation of survival. In one study, only 8 percent were totally unwilling to repeat an ICU experience in order to extend life. Other studies have shown similar results.[42] Beyond that, a majority say they would want such "ordinary" treatment as antibiotics even if they rejected artificially provided nutrition and hydration—though the former is more likely to be needed to sustain their lives than the latter.

What are we to make of those results? Different interpretations are possible, though in general they suggest that people are far more prepared to accept treatment than their prior statements would indicate. The most obvious point to note is that survey questions about what people will want under hypothetical conditions are notoriously unreliable guides to what they will actually do in practice. This has been well known for years by experts in survey research and polling.[43] People sometimes say what they think is acceptable to say, not necessarily what they really believe. Nor can people easily know what they will really want in the distant future, especially when death is a real possibility. There are also other ways to interpret the discrepancy between what people say they want and what they actually get. Some would argue that patients accept livesaving, aggressive treatment mainly because they are induced to do so by doctors; they are swayed or persuaded to give up their own, real, preferences by physicians who have little insight into their needs.[44] That is surely possible, but it is just as plausible to think that patient preferences incline toward the same kind of brinkmanship detectable with physicians. Patients also tend to want to see how close they can come to the border of life and death before being forced to stop treatment.

Not all patients want this, but a large majority do. Since the possibility of some small chance of success is increasingly present because of medical advances, most patients will, then, receive active, life-extending treatment to stave off death. As one physician put it in describing efforts to save an eighty-seven-year-old victim of an auto accident, whose body had been smashed and who remained only semiconscious days later: "He's still hanging in there, going back for his umpteenth orthopedic procedure. The odds of him actually surviving are incredibly slim. But theoretically everything is reversible. So we just trudge along and see what happens."[45] It will be those cases, after the patients' death, that will lead both family members and other medical-staff people to wonder: "Why in the world was he kept alive so long? Why was he given so much useless treatment?" The answer often comes down to a series of subtle, small, incremental steps, none of which actually thwarted patient or family wishes in any obvious fashion, and each of which was based on some hopeful medical possibility, with both the hope and the possibility stimulating each other to the point of folly.

More generally, we fail to realize how profoundly ambivalent most of us are about accepting death, not just because of the threat of death itself, but because we are heirs of the same tradition of technological optimism that has dominated modern medicine. Even if we *say* we can accept death, we believe in our hearts that the sting of death can be medically delayed, that fatalism is itself a source of fatality, that death is a kind of human artifact. No less than physicians have we laypeople come to believe that part of the success of modern medicine stems from a commitment to a zealous use of technology, a zeal no place better expressed than at the margins and against the odds. We believe as a general value that one ought, with spirit, to fight death. We may with all sincerity mean it when we say we do not want clearly useless or futile treatment. But that is not of much help when clinical uncertainty or psychological ambivalence are present; then we may waver, unsure of ourselves. We are all co-conspirators with medicine against death, more than we think.

Why is it so hard to die a tame death? We now see another important reason: to the superheightened uncertainty induced by medicine's promise to help us fight and reject death we can see added a deepened uncertainty about what we should or should not want in our struggles with our mortality.

Why the Past Cannot Be Recaptured

Is a tame death once again possible? Is it desirable? I used the work of Philippe Ariès as my point of departure for two reasons. His historical studies of death left us with a valuable legacy of information and insight into death in earlier times, and reveal what we have lost in the shift to modern death. No less valuable are some of the questions he bequeathed to us, questions that have still to be answered.

Some hesitations are now in order. Ariès's own story about the past is incomplete. It does not pay attention to the pain that marked many earlier deaths, unrelieved by narcotics or analgesics. There were no respirators to relieve the suffocation induced by collapsing lungs, or drugs to control the erratic beat of a heart out of control, or antibiotics to stem gangrene or the torture of spreading bedsores. If the course of dying was usually shorter, it could be and often was more intense in its agonies. A tame death was, it seems, possible and common, but by no means certain; luck and chance played their part. The same consciousness that allowed for a tame death, alert to the end, could also, under less favorable circumstances, make possible an awareness of the pain of a last, fatal, illness.

The price, moreover, of the tame death brought on by the rapid death of an epidemic, common and widespread in earlier centuries, was the devastation of entire families. The cemetery of the early-seventeenth-century Dutch settlers not far from where I live on the Hudson River has one tombstone with the name of five children, all from a single family and all dead within a week of one another. The accompanying tombstone of their parents showed their deaths coming many years later. They could not possibly have used the word "tame" to describe the loss of their children, even if perhaps the children themselves suffered no severe pain in dying. Sometimes entire towns were decimated and whole regions assaulted by disease; and all that on top of already high death rates from ordinary disease and infection. Nor did this kind of widespread death affect bodies only. It could also cause the abandonment of responsible government and medical care. Doctors fled out of fear for their lives, and with them those city fathers responsible for public order. Chaos and despair often followed.

Yet it was the prematurity of those earlier tame deaths that marks the greatest difference between earlier and modern times. When the average life expectancy was not much more than thirty years, tame deaths, though they struck particularly hard at infants and mothers, were easily capable of carrying away people of all ages. Death understandably became familiar in this context. There are no good reasons to want to return to those earlier social and medical conditions that made a certain kind of tame death possible but also allowed death that could, with some frequency, be anything but tame.

We need, nonetheless, to recognize the kind of bargain that has, in effect, been made: we will live longer lives, be better sustained by medical care, in return for which our deaths in old age are more likely to be drawn out and wild. Can we, under these new circumstances, give an answer to a question Ariès posed: "Must we take for granted that it is impossible for our technological culture ever to regain the naive confidence in Destiny which had for so long been shown by simple men when dying?"[46] It is impossible, I believe, even if I wish it could be otherwise. The human ability to modify and manipulate the conditions of death, the uncertain line between life and death, and the absence of a common religious culture all stand in the way of any confident view of "Destiny."

Creating a Peaceful Death

Yet we are not at the end of our resources. There is at the core of the idea of a tame death, and the kind of culture necessary to sustain it, a powerful image, and perhaps a truth: that of a dying that is accepted without overpowering fear and a death that has lost its power to terrorize. I do not mean here to minimize the questions that a tame death can leave with us, whether death should be understood as an evil, and whether a meaning can be given to death. Those questions will remain to shadow all deaths, including tame ones. Nonetheless, there are at least some enduring features of a tame death that we can try to regain, though not in precisely the same form.

I will call this, simply, a "peaceful" death, to signal some changes from the eras that Ariès described, and also to distinguish the difference that modern medicine does and must make in the way we think about what Ariès called a tame death. What must a peaceful death encompass? There is the need to fashion a notion of the self that has, in some sustaining way, come to accept death, a self that understands that control over fate will pass from its hands, that this is precisely what biological death means and must mean. It should also be a death marked by consciousness, by a self-awareness that one is dying, that the end has come—but, even more pointedly, a death marked by self-possession, by a sense that one is ending one's days awake, alert, and physically independent, not as a machine-sustained body or a body that has long ago lost its mind and self-awareness. Equally, it should again be a death in public, by which I mean a time when friends and family draw near, when leave can be taken, when the props and devices of medicine can be put aside save for those meant to palliate and assuage.

In invoking these ideas of a recoverable peaceful death I am not, as it turns out, proposing anything other than what most people seem already to want, and what in fact many people already get. But not all. An accepted death, an alert, conscious death, and a death supported by loving friends and family are ideals now widely espoused. Yet there is great fear that such a death will prove elusive. If a peaceful death is to be possible as a more widespread reality—and, no less important, *believed* to be possible—a fresh interpretation of death will have to be devised and put into place, one now alert to the new conditions of dying. The most central of such conditions is that shaped by medicine itself, the very same medicine that, in its modern scientific form, most directly brought about the demise of the older tame death. That is why I want to distinguish between the older "tame" death and a "peaceful" death. It is a medicine whose most glorious if overweening promise is that of pacifying and modifying mortality. Death is still our common destiny, but how and when that destiny appears has come within the medical grasp—not completely, not perfectly, but there nevertheless. For that reason alone, we cannot regain the "naive confidence in Destiny" that may once have been possible. This does not relieve us of the necessity of understanding how the more complex destiny possible to us may best be realized.

To carry out this task, we must move beyond the domain of medicine alone. What are we to make of nature, of which we are a part and which medicine presumes to work with and to change where possible? Given the power of medical technology to shape and change nature, how are we to understand the powers of that technology and the way, in turn, they lead us to think differently about nature? How, in particular, do those powers lead us to understand the self differently, that self which must now move uneasily and uncertainly between the real and compelling promise of medicine to extend our lives and the realization that, even so, death will still in the end be our destiny?

This profound puzzle cannot fail to be disturbing. It is hard to understand why, since there has been such great progress, we still remain so vulnerable to illness and death. How can we have come so far in medicine, spent so much money on it, have placed such hopes in it, and yet still get sick and die? There is a comfortable answer to this question. It is to attribute that sense of vulnerability to the remaining undone tasks of medical research—all those diseases yet to be cured, those disabilities yet to be overcome.

Yet, ironically and vexingly, whatever progress we achieve seems only to heighten the sense of vulnerability. It is not easy to imagine dying as did Solzhenitsyn's peasant or the Civil War soldier, though in fact such a death still happens more frequently perhaps than people think. Greater medical knowledge, we might recollect, results not only in longer and in many respects healthier lives. It also tells us more knowingly than ever just what continues to threaten our lives. Medical knowledge expands our knowledge of the omnipresence of death, no less than of ways to avert it. That same knowledge tells us with ever-greater precision about our chances of ending our lives with dementia, or languishing frail and dependent in a nursing home, or contracting cancer. It tells us more strikingly than was once the case just what is likely to be the unhappy result in disability if our lives are saved as low-birth-weight babies, or as teenage auto-accident victims, or elderly sufferers from end-stage kidney disease.

We have traded the earlier sense of helplessness and fixed destiny for a heightened sense of choice and control, only to find that we still feel threatened and under siege. As Sigmund Freud aptly expressed it, we are left with "the painful riddle of death, against which no medicine has been found, nor probably will be. With these forces nature rises up against us, majestic, cruel, and inexorable; she brings to our mind once more our weakness and helplessness."[47] Can we achieve as a general rule a peaceful death, but now one that is our own and not a vain attempt to bring back a world that can never exist again? That will not likely be possible unless some further tasks are accomplished. In this chapter I have tried to show that the move to rights and choice as a way out cannot bear the weight placed on it; it is not enough. We bring to our choices a distorted view of nature, one that has affected the practice of medicine and the value assigned to human life in the context of that medicine. It is important to understand those distortions, and to them I now turn.

Chapter 2

STRIPPING DEATH BARE:
THE RECOVERY OF
NATURE

Death has two powerful imaginative roles. It reminds us in the most unmistakable terms that our individual lives will encounter sooner or later a fixed boundary that, whatever our hopes and dreams might be, death will have the last word. Death also reminds us, as members of families and societies, of the passing of the generations, of the bite of social time. Time means that as children we will grow into the adults who manage the world, start families, and make and love friends. That same time moves us into old age, out of power, watching our children come into the strength and place in the world that were once ours. However varied the narratives of human lives, they must all encompass death. All personal stories come to an end. Old families give way to new families. That has been the way of nature.

The ambition of modern medicine has been to do something about that seemingly unalterable fact. It has declared war on death, on the ravages of time, and most of all on the nature that brings them about. It has sought through research to combat the causes of death and constantly to redefine the idea of a premature death. Where a lethal nature once held sway, roughly and unilaterally asserting its force, technological artifact has been brought in to take its place. Medicine has worked to bring nature to heel, to exploit nature itself cleverly to overcome the limits that it seemed to set on our biological lives.

That project has, in its general outline, been a success. Life has been lengthened and death increasingly pushed into old age. People live who would once have died. Yet medicine has failed at one critical point, that of managing the passage between life and death. It does not know, in any reliable technical or emotional way, how to enhance the possibility of a reasonably peaceful death. Part of this failure is inevitable; there will always be some anguish and uncertainty about the coming of death. But more important is the fact that modern medicine has yet to develop a coherent and integrated understanding of the place of death as part of its effort to remake the human biological condition. In its press to master mortality, medicine has come to distort its understanding of nature, a distortion aided and abetted by public expectations, nicely feeding medicine's own confusions. That distortion can be simply stated: medicine has come, in its working research, and often clinical agenda, to look upon death as a correctable biological deficiency. This stance has thus introduced into the practice of medicine and public attitudes a profound and often destructive self-contradiction. We have been left fundamentally uncertain whether death is to be accepted as part of life or rejected as a repairable accident.

Medicine has further compounded the confusion by conflating human action and the independent actions of nature, imputing to human beings an all-encompassing responsibility for death. We know neither whether death as a biological reality ought to be accepted or rejected nor where, in choosing to struggle against death, we should assign responsibility for death when it does occur. We have thereby created a terrible muddle, combining mistakes in self-perception with profound errors about the relationship of medicine and nature. I want in this chapter to explore the latter and try to make plausible contentions that might seem, at first blush, exceedingly strange.

How Medicine Lost Its Way with Nature

In its modern struggle to combat illness and death, medicine came to confuse its power to alter, control, or eliminate disease with its power to banish mortality. At the same time, it has managed to blur the dividing line between human powers and the powers of nature. Before I take on those errors directly, it is necessary to understand how medicine lost its way in understanding nature. In presenting my account, I want to make something clear. When I speak of what "medicine" did, I do so as a shorthand way of referring to the values and ideologies that have historically informed the thinking and practices of the people in medicine, and in this case in the medical sciences in particular. Medicine, that is, does not act independently of the people who practice it. I want to stress, however, that my analysis is not meant to blame medicine. That is beside the point. The underlying logic of medicine is flawed, but the flaw had to go through a long history before becoming evident in all of its implications. This is not a story of "bad" medicine, but of a good medicine that inadvertently came to lose its way.

Let me advance what I believe is a plausible account of the way medicine came to distort its understanding of nature. I will try to offer a likely story, one with three stages. Death was initially understood by human beings as a natural event, as much an inevitability in their lives as the death of every other organic creature. At the same time, death was widely experienced as an evil, as a threat to our desire to live and to our social lives. But it was interpreted as a religious, metaphysical, or psychological evil, not a moral evil. Why was it not, save for murder, a moral evil? Because it was beyond human control, something visited upon us, not caused by us. Historically, there is good evidence that not until the eighteenth century was it even considered part of the duty of physicians to save life.[1] It may have been Francis Bacon who first introduced that idea in an articulate, forceful way. It is a modern notion, and necessarily so: it was not conceivable until doctors could actually preserve life.

The advent of effective medicine, the kind that can save and extend life, changed the perspective on death as an evil, and that is the second stage of the story. As it became increasingly possible to manipulate the conditions of dying, fatalism was rejected and a moral dimension was added. That dimension soon took the form of a simple principle: since death is an evil in human life, we have a moral obligation to use medical means to combat it. What can be done to struggle against death ought to be done. That gradually became the working moral premise of modern scientific medicine, fully supported by religious and secular authority.

Yet, as this new moral era dawned, it was still under the sway of the old view, that death was a natural (if evil) event, for the most part not under human control. Doctors were not considered failures if their patients died. Death still had the upper hand. By the middle of the twentieth century, however, remarkable strides had been made in reducing mortality rates and extending life. Life expectancy has almost doubled over the course of the twentieth century, infant mortality has been radically reduced, and the great majority of people have come to die in old age. By the end of the century, the timing of a majority of deaths was occasioned by a positive decision on the part of physicians to stop treatment.

The control of death seemed at hand. The new demands of morality, to combat death, and the new possibilities of medical technology, which made that a seemingly feasible goal, joined hands to create our present situation, the third stage of the story. As medicine increased its power over death, morality was called upon to increase its demands to struggle against death. The sanctity of human life was taken to require that struggle and, in medical science, to have found its perfect ally. We should not just verbally affirm the value of life. Thanks to medical advances, we can now act. And if we can act to advance the sanctity of life, then we ought to act. The transformation of death from a biological evil to a moral evil as well had been effected. A basic tension between what we *can* do medically and what we *ought* to do morally was created, but this tension put all of the weight on the side of medical activism, the impulse to change and manipulate nature.

How could it have happened? Embedded in the historical changes I have sketched is what I will call the "moral logic" of medical progress. By that phrase I mean the way in which the concept of progress, referring initially only to scientific possibility, comes to take on the force of a moral imperative: what can be known ought to be known, and what can be done ought to be done.

To make clear what I mean by this moral logic, we might first recollect a key feature of the modern history of medical thought. Though in many ways a conservative discipline, medicine gradually became by the end of the nineteenth century one of the most enthusiastic acolytes of the Enlightenment idea of progress. Through basic biological knowledge and its clinical application, medicine can constantly advance the frontier of human health: the possibilities of progress are unlimited. This is now an article of faith in modern medicine, well supported by the evidence of past success and the reasonable likelihood of constant continuing success. The scope of progress includes not only increased knowledge and technological skills. It permeates as well our notions of the ends of medicine, the meaning of health, and the ways in which human lives can be led. In that sense, the idea of progress is an enormous intensifier, the deepest animating force, of the historical stages earlier described.

What is the moral logic of this process? The scientific imperative of progress, part of the idea of medical science, is broadened to include a moral imperative: if we do not pursue the conquest of disease, we are open to moral blame. People will die who need not die. If we do not use our newly available technologies to save lives, we can be held accountable for the loss of those lives. The hidden, but hardly arcane, premise here is that we have a duty to relieve suffering and to save life. If medical progress makes that possible, then we are *obliged* to pursue it. The pursuit, say, of the Genome Project, the mapping of the human genome, is more than scientifically exciting and thus desirable. Its promise of the cure or relief of genetic disease creates a powerful moral demand: pursue this project or be forever guilty of abandoning those in need. If we believe it morally necessary to save, through heart transplants, the lives of those who would otherwise die, how can we not pursue the artificial heart to save those who are not candidates for transplants?

The Disappearance of Nature

Stimulated by that moral activism, the scientific effort to understand and control the causes of illness and death has progressed at a dazzling pace. Yet in the process some puzzles have emerged. Is death still a reality only because we have not been clever enough to overcome it? Is it perhaps not fixed and permanent, as once thought, but plastic and remediable? The death of babies in infancy was once thought a law of nature. That law has been repealed—almost repealed, anyway—by biological knowledge and neonatal technology. If each and every death is caused by a specific disease or condition, why not go after and eradicate them? Eventually there will be none left. Who says we are slaves of nature?

Who says, for that matter, that there is even a nature distinct from our human powers and creations? Is there a *real* nature out there? The idea of nature as an alien, independent reality has a long history, going back to the animism of primitive tribes for whom nature was filled with gods and demons, alive and active in the world. Modern history has seen two great changes. The first, from the Greeks forward, saw the removal of the gods and spirits from nature, thus rendering it inert—the disenchantment of nature; and then, through science stimulated by the Enlightenment, the discovery of the laws and dynamic of a now impersonal, but not necessarily unchangeable, nature. Bacon's famous remark that knowledge is power—the power to change nature—has long stood as emblematic of this shift.

The second great change, more recent, has been to ask a new question: does it any longer make sense to think of nature as having some essence and independent reality of its own, distinct from human agency, imagination, and interpretation?[2] Should not our own actions in changing the world count as part of nature? And should not our technical creations be understood now as a part of nature? If even our observations of nature change that which we observe, as now widely believed, or our theories about nature themselves modify that which they would explain, how can we find a line between ourselves and nature? Why should we even think there is one?

The animistic spirits of the primitives, once in animals and trees and planets, have now, so to speak, been transferred to ourselves. It is our agency, our action, that makes nature what it is, or (more to the point) what we take it to be, a nature now to be understood as a creative interpretation, a work of imaginative artifice, rather than a separable reality simply to be described as it is. As the late O. B. Hardison nicely put it, "If science is a human creation, we have caught the mind in the very act of swallowing the world, which is another way we have witnessed nature in the process of disappearing."[3]

Faced with death, we may be tempted to dismiss that way of thinking about nature as romantic and fanciful. Nature has not disappeared at all, it might be replied; its bite has simply been softened a bit. But I want to suggest that the idea of a vanished nature, replaced by human art and scientific artifice, is powerfully alive, though often hidden below the surface.

Consider the following commonplace events:

• Doctors routinely resist turning off respirators and other life-sustaining machines with irreversibly dying patients, because they experience their action as tantamount to killing the patient. Those patients, they believe, will die from their action in stopping the machine, rather than from the underlying disease. Even if they believe their action morally justifiable, they may still feel lingering guilt that they caused the death.

• Physicians are commonly more willing not to start a treatment in the first place with a dying person (withholding treatment) than to end that treatment once started (withdrawing treatment). In the former case, they think the disease will be responsible for the death. In the latter, they believe it will be their decision to stop that will end the life.

• Many nurses and doctors are reluctant, and sometimes refuse, to accept decisions to stop artificial nutrition with dying patients or those in a persistent vegetative state. Their reasoning is that the patient will then be starved to death because of their omission, construed as an action (stopping) which terminates feeding.

• Research advocates often argue that a failure to allocate money to the search for a cure of a lethal disease (e.g., AIDS, breast cancer, Alzheimer's disease) will leave the blood of the continuing deaths on the hands of those who deny the money.

• Many liberal philosophers and theologians contend that there is no moral difference between allowing a patient to die from an underlying disease and killing that patient directly by, say, an injection. They conclude that, if allowing a patient to die is acceptable, it is equally acceptable morally, and often more merciful, to kill that patient directly.

• Numerous conservative philosophers and theologians believe that in many circumstances allowing a patient to die by stopping treatment is a discreet way of intentionally killing that patient. Therefore, they conclude, if directly killing a patient is morally wrong, it can be equally wrong to intentionally allow a patient to die who could be saved by "ordinary" treatment.

• Many physicians believe that a patient is dying not because of what is happening to his body but because there are no further medical or technological strategies available to keep the patient alive. Death is not construed as an inevitable biological denouement but as a medical failure. "The patient," an important study found, "is not even defined as dying until the clinicians determine there are no further interventions they can make that will improve the patient's condition."[4] Death has been moved out of nature into the realm of human responsibility.

Nature and Human Action: The Vanishing Line

What is the common feature in each of these situations? It is an interpretation of where the line between human actions and causes, on the one hand, and the causes and forces of an independent nature, on the other, is to be found. Or whether there any longer even exists such a line. Long before the advent of modern medicine, to be sure, questions of the moral and legal difference between acts of commission and omission, killing and allowing to die, acting and refraining from acting, were debated. There have always been serious problems in making such distinctions. If, through laziness, I allowed a child to drown whom I could have rescued, did I cause that child's death? If, as a landlord, I fail to repair defective wiring and a fatal fire results, am I responsible for those fatalities? If I neglect to warn someone of a hazard in the road ahead, is the ensuing accident my fault?

Those are old and familiar puzzles, each of them bearing on the relationship between human and natural causes. Law and custom have, for the most part, found answers to them, as the extensive literature and case law on negligence shows. But those long-standing problems have taken on a new dimension in the instance of death and modern medicine. At one time, when medicine could do little to alter the course of biological nature, it was comparatively easy to say that a patient died of her disease, not of any failure or omission on the part of the physician. When physicians could do nothing, they could hardly be held accountable for what happened to their patients. The inexorable forces of nature killed people: accidents, disease, and aging.

Everything changed once medical action could make a difference. A patient can live if the right drug is prescribed, but die if a mistake is made. Before the discovery of insulin, diabetes killed people. They can now also be killed, so moral and social convention has it, by a culpable failure not to give them insulin. Even so, for a long time a distinction was made between death as the result of "natural causes" and death that came about because of human failure, mistakes, or omissions. Disease was still understood to be the physical cause of death in those cases, but doctors could be held responsible for their failure to control that cause appropriately, if it was possible for them to do so. It was, in short, possible to distinguish between physical *causality* (the impersonal, independent force of biological processes) and moral *culpability* (the responsibility of human beings for their actions, or omissions, in response to those processes).

Under this traditional interpretation, if I fail to give a child his shot of insulin and the child dies, I am morally at fault, *culpable* for my omitted act. But the actual *cause* of his death will be diabetes. I wrongly allowed his death to take place, but that death could not have happened had there not been an underlying physical deficiency; and it is that deficiency which is the actual cause of death.

This way of thinking is gradually disappearing—mistakenly, in my belief—and with it vanishes the concept of nature that made such distinctions plausible and meaningful. Some hold that to hang on to such distinctions is a form of self-deception, helping to make physicians and others feel better about the lives they take. We like, it is said, to pretend to ourselves that nature does the killing, not ourselves. As a result of such changes and interpretations, culpability and causality have become increasingly muddled, intertwined in a tangled knot whose separate strands can hardly be discovered any longer.

What has emerged as a result? It is the powerful tendency to attribute *everything* that happens to human agency, what we do and what we fail to do, our omissions and our commissions. That is the salient feature of the various "commonplace events" I noted above. They bespeak in their different ways the loss of a conviction that nature still has its own separate ways, that it exists apart from us. Our actions have come instead to be of the greatest consequence. More than that, even our omissions have a force and result every bit as powerful as what we do; and what we do has the same force and status that was once reserved to nature alone.

The overturning of the dominance of nature is now complete.

Where once we human beings as moral agents stood helpless in the face of nature, whose workings were outside the range of our responsibility, now everything is in some sense thought to be our responsibility. Causality and culpability have been collapsed together. The doctor who cannot save a patient faults her lack of skill, or medicine's lack of a cure; it might have been otherwise. The nurse who watches a feeding tube removed from a hopelessly ill patient thinks the patient is being killed by the removal, not by the disease that made the tube necessary. The euthanasia advocate holds that, by our adherence to a fictitious notion of "allowing to die" from an underlying disease, we willfully condemn a patient to needless suffering; direct killing would be more merciful, and the act of killing no different in any case from that of allowing to die. The euthanasia opponent, wary of badly motivated people using nature and its ways as an excuse, comes to see culpability in the movement to make allowing to die easier. There is as much potential fault there as in outright killing, only it is more hypocritical and hidden.

Mortality: Blaming the Victim

I want to call this general pattern, discernible in so many areas of medicine and medical morality, "technological monism." By this term I mean the tendency to erase the difference between human action as a cause of what happens in the world, and independent, natural biological processes, those old-fashioned causes of disease and death. It is nothing less than an ingenious way of blaming the victim, as if death itself were now our fault, the result of human choices, not the independent workings of nature.

That is how nature, to use O. B. Hardison's nice phrase, "disappears through the skylight" in the medical realm, now replaced by what we as human beings do or do not do.[5] Whatever is left of nature has become only a facilitating medium for our acts and works. It is the stuff—malleable, plastic, workable, transformable, and controlled by no inherent essence—out of which they are fashioned. What we used to call the "brute reality" of nature has now been swallowed up in the medical construction of a new reality, now our creation and, most important, our full and unavoidable responsibility.

Yet we have, in the process of this disappearance of nature, created a new and tyrannical problem. We have done nothing less than to make mortality itself our fault, our responsibility. By making humans responsible for everything, and making it irrelevant whether they act by commission or omission, we have created an impossibly heavy and unbearable burden. How can that have happened? Very easily. If each individual death is understood as in principle a medical and thus a *human* causal and moral responsibility, then the biological status of death itself is rendered inherently uncertain. It continues to reign, but accidentally and contingently, not necessarily. We are still asked, plaintively, to "accept death." Why, however, should anyone accept that which need not be?

This might simply be a burdensome paradox, not inherently tyrannical. The real tyranny comes in deciding how and when to use available medical technology, and in deciding whether to develop still more technology. The use of technology is ordinarily the way, in modern medicine, that action is carried out: to give a pill, to cut out a cancerous tumor, or to use a machine to support respiration. With an ethos of technological monism, all meaningful actions—and thus all meaningful causes—are technological, whether technological acts or technological omissions. What nature does, its underlying natural causes and pathologies, becomes irrelevant. No death is "natural" any longer—the word becomes meaningless—no natural cause necessarily determinative, no pathology fatal unless failure to deploy a technology makes it so. Perhaps it was an act of desperation in response to this disappearance of nature that the early "living will" legislation was often introduced as an effort to achieve a "natural" death and the legislative bills themselves called "natural death" acts. In other words, the public discussion of death came to presuppose that death is no longer natural; only a new kind of patient choice could make it so once again.

The tyranny once attributed to a fixed, immutable nature, beyond human power or control, has now been transferred to the human realm. The power of technology imposes the new determinism. Whereas nature once decided who would live or die, our technological capacities have come to play that role. Whereas once nature could be faulted for bringing death, it has become our choice to use or not use a technology that will bear the responsibility.

But why do I call this the "new determinism"? Do we not retain voluntary control over the technologies? That old, external, independent nature was not our creature; the new technologies are. In one sense, all that is surely true. Machines can be and are turned off, drugs omitted, operations not undertaken. But, in another sense, it is far less true. The change from a dualistic world where physical cause and moral culpability could be kept separate to one where they are collapsed creates an entirely different context for choice, one far more constricting than might seem the case.

Prisoners of Choice

In the former world of nature, some acts and events were our responsibility, others not, and mostly not. In the new world of vanished nature, they are *all* our responsibility. Moreover, they are all our responsibility in the context of powerful and evolving technologies, which leave increasingly unclear the lines between living and dying, and impose their own imperative for use precisely because they do so. Where nature was, human choice is. Where choice is, technology is. Where technology is, choice is transformed. The illusion has been fostered that we are now as gods, the cause (real or potential) of all that is, and morally responsible for whatever is or could be. It is not as if we do not know better. It is that we have stopped acting on what we know.

The results are strange, often bizarre. In the name of the sanctity of life, many who would consider themselves conservative and supporters of traditional religious values are forced into a slavery to medical possibilities, held in thrall by the false god of technology. The value of life is in practice defined, not by religious or moral principles as traditionalists wish, but by technical capacities. The Roman Catholic teaching on the distinction between ordinary and extraordinary treatment is a good example of this. The main point of the original distinction was not, as commonly thought, to distinguish between technically simple and technically complicated medical procedures. It was meant instead to underscore the difference between those treatments that impose no great burden of pain, cost, or inconvenience on a patient and those that do. But conservative supporters of the distinction now argue that it is the burden of *treatment*—will it or will it not, for instance, cause great pain?—that is at stake in the distinction, not the burden of the life that will result from the treatment. Repudiated, therefore, is the idea that quality-of-life judgments should or can morally be made.[6]

The strange problem that results, however, is that, as long as a treatment itself is beneficial in sustaining life and not burdensome, there is an obligation to use it. It must be used, it would seem, even if the result is to extend a life in great pain, or severe dementia, or permanent unconsciousness. If an inexpensive antibiotic, itself a painless treatment, can extend life, then it must be used, regardless of what the life thus preserved may be like. It is ordinary treatment, and it is nonburdensome treatment; therefore it must be used, even if it leaves the patient as a person worse off than before, and even if it enhances the likelihood that a later death will be worse than the one averted.

The outcome of this reasoning is as clear a case of slavery to technology as can be found, and all the more ironically hazardous to a peaceful death. Medicine will increasingly become far more skilled at developing nonburdensome treatments than treatments that have a positive effect on the quality of human lives. Supporters of the view that only treatment burdens should count have been beguiled into acting as if a failure to use technology is tantamount to deliberate killing, an act inimical to life's sanctity. The logic of their position will force them to go wherever technology goes. Machines can only with reluctance be turned off, feeding tubes routinely inserted and then never or hardly ever pulled, ordinary nonburdensome antibiotics never withheld, and all efforts to omit treatment regarded with a sometimes extreme wariness. I am not claiming a strict logical entailment here, as if those making the treatment-burden distinction cannot say no to technology, or draw lines. I am instead saying that the required weight of proof, on the one hand, and the level of suspicion about motives, on the other, are so great that the practical consequences will tend to be devastating to even legitimate efforts to allow patients to die. Though they have not directly been part of this technical debate, its flavor and substance is reflected in the extreme reluctance of physicians to omit the use of simple lifesaving therapeutics, even if the life saved will be terrible.

There is no less of a problem at the other end of the ideological spectrum. Those seeking a liberalization of older rules and mores seize upon the erasure of the distinction between nature and human agency as the occasion for a final and total control of human life through euthanasia and assisted suicide: autonomy triumphant, suffering banished, wasted money saved. They, no less than their opponents, have been tyrannized, this time by the idea that, if they can act, they must act. Disease must be banished to avert suffering; and if suffering cannot be banished that way, then it ought to be eliminated by euthanasia. To refuse to act decisively in the face of suffering, with direct killing if necessary, is to be responsible for it.

Recovering Nature

The emergence of technological monism, a consequence of a vanishing nature, helps make clear the dilemma we face. If we allow that monism to hold sway, our medical morality is almost certain to be controlled by technology, leaving little middle ground between a fear ever to stop using it, or a compulsion to stop it only by a dangerous practice of euthanasia. Yet it will not be easy to find a standard of moral judgment by a simple return to the old nature. With technology itself now a part of reality, nature pure and simple will not provide clear messages about when death is inevitable, or when a decent quality of life can no longer be maintained, or when treatment is futile. In that respect, technology has made a great difference. We cannot return to a premodern world, nor should we want to.

Yet we must restore nature to put the human responsibility for death into a more fitting focus. We need a plausible and useful interpretation of nature, one free of the conceit that nature has disappeared, and free in particular of its medical corollary, a technological monism that can find no boundary to human responsibility for life and death. A peaceful death can never be ours if we let that view hold sway. How might a restoration be sought? I shall propose a partial answer to this question in this chapter, then round out my approach in chapter 5.

The necessary place to begin is with three fundamental errors that have made their way into common thinking, both medical and lay. Taken together, they tell the story of the way nature has been distorted. The first is the pervasive belief that, *although death may be inevitable, none of the medical causes of death need be accepted; all are in principle curable.* The second error is the widespread conviction that *there is, in the end, no fundamental moral difference between killing a person and allowing a person to die.* The third error is that *a commitment to the sanctity of human life is best expressed and pursued through medical science and technological aggressiveness against death.* The first of these errors helps to explain why those trained in modern medicine can claim to accept death as part of biological life yet, in practice, find it so difficult to allow a patient to die from a particular disease—the only way a patient can die. The second error helps illuminate why, for some, allowing to die can seem an overwhelming moral burden (if it is likened to killing) and, for others, why killing may come to be as acceptable as allowing to die. The third error helps to make clear why a commitment to the value and sanctity of life has often ended in a captivity to technology, which is tacitly allowed to dictate moral standards.

Accidental Disease, Necessary Death

"Death," Dr. Otto Guttentag told me well over two decades ago, "has no place in modern medicine. Only pathologists take death seriously."[7] I thought at first he was simply making a joke. He was not. Death is for the most part absent in modern textbooks of medicine, where the science of the field is collected and distilled for use in practice. Except for a place in the (usually minor) medical-ethics part of a medical-school curriculum, it has no significant place in the training of physicians either. I was once able to get an audience of medical-school educators to agree, albeit sheepishly, that there was probably more discussion of making decisions about dying patients on daytime soap operas (where it is a favorite theme) than in their classrooms. Why? Because death has no meaningful place within the rationale and goals of scientific medicine, whose latent purpose is to overcome death. I specify here "scientific medicine," by which I mean the ideology, and the particular methods of research and treatment, that constitute the heart of modern medicine. Clinical medicine, where the move must be made from science to the bedside, and where uncertainty and ambiguity are taken to be part of the practice, is a different matter. The goal of scientific-research medicine is to overcome disease, to overcome that which brings illness and death. Death is the greatest enemy, and disease its army. There is no important human disease, or class of diseases, that the National Institutes of Health are not seeking to cure and eliminate. Grant money is available to fight all of them. There are, by contrast, *no* scientific-research grants available from that institution to help us better understand how to live with the mortality caused by those diseases. Death thus remains curiously outside scientific medicine altogether. It is the unspeakable opponent.

How could this have happened? Medicine, I believe, has implicitly defined its central purpose as an all-out fight against death. Yet what is true of the scientific enterprise of medicine is by no means equally true of clinical medicine at the bedside, even if the latter has been powerfully influenced by it and has come to encourage it. Every physician knows that patients die, that for every illness for which a cure can be found for a patient this time, there will be one, at a later time, that will not admit of a cure. There will always be a last, fatal illness for every patient, an illness that will be caused by a specific disease. For all the obviousness of that perception, however, scientific medicine has managed to keep it at bay in its own research logic. Who says patients have to die? Who says that the causes of death cannot be defeated? Death remains the enemy. Clinicians have to cope with it; they know well enough that death can sometimes be welcomed. But the tension between scientific medicine, meant to represent the highest ideals and loftiest intellectual elegance of the field, and clinical medicine is powerful. Scientific medicine, with its war on death and disease, is also at war with clinical medicine, which must make its daily peace with them.

The deepest part of this tension is not just in how it creates a battle in the heart of a physician (or a patient's family), but in its understanding of the connection between death and disease. Death is understood well enough to be a biological necessity, a part of nature, even if that point is not made in medical textbooks. But every cause of death is taken to be contingent, a matter of chance. By "contingent" and "chance" I mean that it need not exist, that there is *in principle* and in medical *theory* no reason why any *particular* disease cannot be overcome. Death is in some sense biologically programmed, but not particular causes of death. Just as smallpox was eliminated, and diphtheria and typhoid and typhus all but eradicated, so cancer and Alzheimer's can also be done away with. This is the abiding faith

of scientific medicine. No cause of death has been declared beyond hope; none could be. All of the known causes of death
can, in principle, be picked off, one by one. All of the wars
against disease can eventually be won, not only those that kill
us but also those that weigh down our aging.

Where does this leave our mortality? In a strange place, both
real and unreal at the same time. It is real in the sense that there
is now, and will always be, death, and for every living being.
Mortality as part of our fate lies undisturbed by progress. No one
has ever been able to show how, in theory or practice, it could
be entirely eliminated from human existence. Yet that same
mortality becomes unreal in the sense that no particular, concrete
cause of death need exist. Death in general is inevitable, but
death in particular is contingent. Every possible cause of death
could be seen as a piece of bad luck: an accident that could have
been prevented, a cancer or an infection that might have been
caught in time, a disease that would not have killed me if I had
contracted it years from now, when a treatment would be available, even a genetic disease that might have been avoided had
early screening been available to my parents. In my parents'
generation, the old died of "natural causes." No such luck any
longer.

The cure for this problem is as simple as the puzzle that gives
rise to it in the first place. How can mortality be our fate if there
is, in principle, no specific cause of death that does not admit
of a potential cure? The answer is obvious and thus easily overlooked: when one disease has been cured, another will take its
place. Mortality works backward, so to speak. We will die of
something, because our bodies will age and be unable to renew
themselves. If one thing does not get us, another will. We will
and must die of some disease—if not those at present on the
horizon, which may be cured, then those that will take their
place. Unless it could be shown scientifically that there is some
imaginable final disease that, when overcome, would admit of
or allow no successor disease, death must remain our lot.

Killing and Allowing to Die

No philosophical puzzle is so pervasive in modern medicine as the moral evaluation of the line, if any, between acts of commission and omission, between human agency and natural causes.[8] If we accept the idea that nature has disappeared, that line disappears as well. The distinction between killing a person and allowing that person to die, it has been argued, should be done away with. I want to contend, on the contrary, that the long-standing, traditional moral distinction retains its validity. There is and will always remain a fundamental difference between what nature does to us and what we do to one another. No better evidence of the power of the idea of a vanishing nature can be found than in the enthusiasm to scrap that difference.

Why do some want to reject it? I can do no better than to quote directly the words of one of the most articulate critics of the distinction, James Rachels: "The bare difference between killing and letting die does not, in itself, make a moral difference. If a doctor lets a patient die for humane reasons, he is in the same moral position as if he had given the patient a lethal injection for humane reasons. If his decision was wrong—if, for example, the patient's illness was in fact curable—the decision would be equally regrettable no matter which method was used to carry it out. And if the doctor's decision was the right one, the method used was not in itself important."[9] In criticism of a statement by the American Medical Association upholding the traditional distinction, Rachels goes on to say that the statement is wrong in denying "that the cessation of treatment is the intentional termination of life. . . . Of course it is exactly that, and if it were not, there would be no point to it."[10]

There are three mistakes here, all of which stem from what I believe to be Rachels' implicit, but erroneous, understanding of nature. For some purposes, it is surely the case that the "bare difference" is irrelevant: if our *only* concern is to specify whether a doctor's commissions or omissions are morally culpable. A doctor can wrongfully, whether through negligence or intent, allow a patient to die—that is, allow a disease to take its lethal course when, morally speaking, it should have been stopped. But if we ask about the larger significance of the difference between killing and letting die, some important considerations emerge.

The first is that, as a reality of nature, killing and letting die are causally different. "Letting die" is only physically possible if there is some underlying disease that will serve as the cause of death. Put me on a respirator now, when I am in good health, and nothing whatever will happen if it is turned off. I cannot be "allowed to die" by having a respirator turned off if I have healthy lungs. It is wholly different, however, if a doctor gives me a muscle-relaxing injection that will paralyze my lungs. Healthy or not, those lungs will cease to function and I will die. That is what it means to "kill" someone as distinguished from "letting" someone die. Put more formally, there must be an underlying fatal pathology if allowing to die is even possible. Killing, by contrast, provides its own fatal pathology. Nothing but the action of the doctor giving the lethal injection is necessary to bring about death.

Though the result of killing and allowing to die may be the same in one way—a patient is dead in either case—that hardly means that the causal difference between the two incidents is morally irrelevant. Here is Rachels' second mistake: to assume that the intention in letting die is ordinarily the same as in killing, that is, to make a person dead. It is certainly the case that we *might* intend someone's death and turn off a machine to bring that about. But it is equally the case, and far more common in ordinary medical practice, that patients are allowed to die because of a judgment that it no longer makes sense, medically or morally or both, to continue life-extending treatment. Doctors have long stopped treating patients when their skills and art run out. There is no reason to think that, as a rule, it is because their intentional goal is to make people die.

There are two issues to be distinguished here. One of them is what justifies, medically and morally, saying that it no longer makes sense to continue life-extending treatment? The other is the meaning of that judgment when it is used to stop life-extending treatment. It will be sufficient here to say that, once a judgment has been reached about futility, it is considered acceptable by long-standing medical tradition to stop treatment. Doctors ought not to do that which it is useless to do. Such actions would be a misuse of their skills and training, a kind of mockery of their vocation. What, however, is the *meaning* of a judgment of futility, and what intention is expressed when it is acted upon? It is not, and never has been in the generality of cases, a judgment that a patient *ought* to be dead, or would be better off dead. It is not principally a judgment about a patient's life at all. It is, instead, a judgment about the limits of medical skills in providing further patient benefit. It is a way of saying that, because the limits of those skills have been reached, the patient may be allowed to die.

To call those judgments, and the ensuing omission of treatment, "intending" death distorts what actually happens. Some analogies will make this evident. In running a race I see I cannot win, would I be accused of *intending* to lose if I slow up? Or, if I stop shoveling my driveway in a heavy snowstorm because I cannot keep up with it, am I thereby *intending* a driveway full of snow? Ordinarily, we might understand that, if we see that a certain result is a necessary part of the action we intend, we can be said to intend that result (even if we do not want it). Hence, it is common to hold people responsible for what their actions bring about, even if they do not directly will that result.

But this logic does not apply in the case of the dying patient. Since death is biologically inevitable sooner or later, not a consequence of our actions but outside of them, we can hardly be said to "intend" death when we admit we can no longer stop it. Since mortality is our fate, biologically given, at some point treatment must of necessity no longer work to keep us alive. However many successful treatments we undergo, there will always be one, the last one, that fails. That a doctor may keep a patient going for another day or so, but thinks it pointless to prolong the process, does not amount to "intending" death either. The only intention is to stop a pointless action, and, put positively, to affirm the ultimate power of nature, over which we have limited control. Doctors treat patients in the first place because they want to help them, to make them well again. They ordinarily stop treating them when nothing more of value can be done, not because they want or intend them to be dead.

Nowhere is the harmful force of technological monism more potent than in the assumptions about causality and intention that lie behind the belief that to stop useless treatment is to intend death. It is, once again, to conflate human action and natural events, the former swallowing the latter. Not only are doctors made responsible for the omitted treatment that allows death to occur, they are also—as if they are gods—said to intend what nature once wrought. It is a way of thinking that makes medicine the perfect prisoner of its powers, which now encompass actions and intentions.

Rachels' third mistake is to think that the method by which a physician brings about a patient's death is "not in itself important." Yet it is, and for an obvious reason. With "letting die," it is the disease that causes the patient's death, not the doctor; and the doctor's traditional stance of refusing to kill patients has not been changed. In the case of killing, doctors become the cause of death. That shift erases the long-established moral rule against killing by doctors, and also introduces a new justification for killing, that of relieving suffering. Even if one agrees with such a change, can it really be characterized as "not in itself important"? Nothing less than the meaning and goals of medicine is at stake.

I do not want to deny that physicians can wrongly allow patients to die, and thus be culpable for that death. That is why it is understandable to speak colloquially of a doctor's "killing" a patient if treatment is wrongfully stopped. This linguistic convention allows us to place the doctor in the same moral category as those who directly kill others; thus we express the strongest possible moral condemnation. But it is not *literally* the case that the doctor kills. Only the underlying disease can accomplish the necessary condition for death to occur when treatment is stopped.

Why place such a heavy emphasis on the *literal* cause of death? What difference does that make? One reason is that our psychological capacity to keep natural causes clearly before our eyes offers the first line of defense against the delusional force of the idea of a vanishing nature and an increasingly omnipotent human action. It is a vivid, because true, way of reminding ourselves that a physical nature exists out there apart from our actions. Death is not vanishing from nature. It is still a hard and fast part of all biological life. Everyone dies. There always was death, and there is still death.

We did not invent death, and we cannot make it disappear. To collapse causality and culpability, to treat nature as if it had now become dispensable in our moral reckoning, has two harmful, though paradoxical, effects. It reinforces the cultural predilection to deny death altogether, hiding death from sight: if nature has disappeared, so has death. Yet it magnifies into a monstrosity the human responsibility for death. If nature has disappeared, then whatever happens or fails to happen is our human fault. Neither of those alternatives is sensible or tolerable.

There is a no less important reason to keep clear the difference between causality and culpability. That distinction helps to make evident the extent to which moral norms and rules pertinent to death and the treatment of patients have come with time to be laid over, and thus to obscure, a base of natural causation. I mean by that claim simply to make visible the fact that, in dealing with death, human beings have superimposed upon natural causation a web of morality, but so gradually and subtly that the line between nature and morality is blurred. That in turn sets the stage for the technological monism that would make us directly responsible for the deaths that follow all failures to use technology.

The debate about the cessation of artificial nutrition and hydration illustrates the confusions that technological monism has introduced. [11] Some liberals and many conservatives believe that the stopping of such treatment is the moral equivalent of killing the patient. The former think it acceptable to do so—not all killings are morally wrong—whereas the latter consider it mistaken, indeed a cruel starving to death. Both, I have come to believe, are wrong. If an inability to take food and water by mouth is the ordinary concomitant of a terminal illness—as it has been since time immemorial—that should be understood as a symptom (not always certain, of course) of a terminal condition, one way the dying body shuts down its key systems. That circumstance was never, until recently, described as a patient's "starving" to death, which connotes a violent, painful death. The cause of death was understood to be the underlying disease, and the inability to take nourishment by mouth a symptomatic way the deadly disease manifested itself. Indeed, the inability to take food and water itself helped to induce the final, usually gentle, coma. It led to a peaceful, not a violent, death.

All that changed with the advent of widespread means of providing artificial hydration and nutrition. Whereas those means had initially been used to provide a temporary medical bridge for postsurgery patients, a short-term technical treatment, they came increasingly to be used with patients who were unable to take food and water by mouth. Once that practice became routine, it was no longer thought of as "treatment." We quickly forgot that dying had commonly been preceded in the past by a natural inability to eat and take water—"natural" in the sense that it was a regular corollary of more general organ failure. Soon—in a period of less than twenty years, between 1970 and 1990—a whole new category of morally required treatment was created. The upshot was almost foreordained: to stop this new treatment would be to "cause" the death of the patient, and would thus be unacceptable morally. A whole new moral rule had been introduced, superimposed upon the underlying pathological process. What is important to see, however, is that, though a new moral rule, it was one disguised as a statement about nature and the causes of death. Where once nature had killed people by robbing their bodies of the capacity to take nutrition, now the blame has been shifted to the human beings who fail to provide artificial nutrition. It is they, and not the nature that had done the same for thousands of years, who are at fault. This way of reasoning is as nice a case of technological monism as one could ask for.

Creating a Moral Overlay

Let me try to make my argument here a bit clearer. In their discussion of the distinction between omission and commission in the law, the legal scholars H. L. A. Hart and Tony Honoré argue that over time human habits, customs, and conventions have been developed to counteract the harm that results when we fail to intervene in potentially harmful natural events. "These have," they write, "become a 'second nature' and so a second 'norm.' "[12] We can thus say, as common language allows, that a doctor "killed" a patient by his negligent failure to put a suffocating patient on a respirator in a timely fashion. But this way of speaking reflects a moral convention superimposed upon nature, a function of the fact that a moral rule has been developed over time that would hold doctors responsible for *certain* omissions on their part, those that we judge to be wrongful omissions. As long as we understand that it is the created *moral rule* about a physician's obligations, not some judgment on the natural state of affairs, that leads us to speak as if it is the doctor's omission that "kills" the patient, there is no problem. We go wrong, however, when we think that the physician literally caused the death. The death results from the underlying disease, which is the only reason the doctor's omission would make any difference in the outcome. It is only our historically created, humanly devised moral rule about the moral responsibility of physicians that allows us to speak of a doctor's "killing" a patient.

Consider an analogy. If I come across a dying wild animal while on a walk in the woods, it can be said that the animal is dying of "natural causes" and that I have no moral responsibility to save its life. I have no culpability for the causal condition that brought the animal to death's door, or for my failure to attempt to save its life. Our moral rules and conventions have not posited any duty to save dying wild animals. If, by contrast, I come across my neighbor's child dying in the woods from some similar natural cause, whether a disease or an accident, I would be held culpable if I ignored him. Our moral rules and conventions require that I come to his aid. Someone could plausibly accuse me of "killing" the child if, through laziness or indifference, I passed him by. Yet note that the only difference between these two events lies, not in the underlying physical causes that bring death to the animal and the child, but in the moral rules we have superimposed upon those events. I would not be accused of killing the animal, whereas I could be accused of killing the child. Yet the act of omission—the failure to intervene in the natural chain of events—would be exactly the same. The only difference lies in the different moral rules developed to judge the omission.

Nature has not disappeared at all. Since death's ultimate domination is as hard and fast as ever, human beings bear only a limited responsibility for death. We may be held morally responsible for death *only* to the extent that we have erected upon nature a set of moral rules and principles to govern our conduct in manipulating the biology of illness and death. Technological monism—the compulsion to use technology out of a fear that failure to use it makes us responsible for the ensuing death—can only be combated by noting the superstructure of moral rules. We created them and we can change them. More to the point, it is a delusion to think that, because we now have a socially constructed edifice of moral rules and the power to manipulate death by means of technology we have thereby become responsible for death, as if death were now our medical artifact rather than what it still is, an independent biological reality.

The Sanctity of Life and the Technological Imperative

The fear of death and the judgment that death can be an evil seem to provide reason enough to struggle against it. Yet we know from the cruelties of wars, pogroms, and political repressions, or from the more mundane atrocities of our own civilized institutions, that it is easy to become insensitive to death, even to glorify it. No civilized society has been able to depend upon an instinctual fear of death alone to provide the social checks necessary to control violence or to provide a positive impetus to respect life. That has required specific moral rules and commandments, legal sanctions, and the instilling of virtues and habits designed to promote the protection of life. It has required, above all, a positive affirmation of the value of life, not only an invocation of the fear of death. In such concepts as the sanctity of life, or the dignity of individual life, that affirmation has found expression.

Yet with the advent and advance of scientific medicine and other powers to control and modify nature, there has been a profound ambiguity about these efforts. Should death from natural causes and forces outside of human agency—disease, accidents, calamities—be understood as evil in the same sense and to the same degree as deaths caused by human acts? If death is an evil, and life a good, should death by cancer be considered as being as wrong as death by murder? If it is reasonable for a society to seek to avoid even one murder, is it equally reasonable for it to consider even one death by cancer too many?

No. The ultimate evil of death lies in its manifestation of our human limits and finitude. It is a mistake to think that such finitude is best fought by an embrace of medical progress and the forestalling of death. The enlistment of that progress in an unlimited struggle against death from disease is a basic error. If it is of our nature as biological creatures to die, one manifestation of our finitude but not the only one by any means, then it is foolish to think death can be overcome by medical science. It is even more misguided to believe that we do honor to life, or express our distaste for the phenomenon of death, by always seeing death as the enemy. It is *an* enemy, but not *the* enemy. *The* enemy is our finitude, our ultimately unrequited longing for more than we have. We resist death because it stands as a consummate nasty symbol, and the great wrenching finale, of a life that is endlessly marked by limits, boundaries, fences, and contradictions. I will call the "medical fallacy" the belief that in medicine we have found the appropriate cure for our finitude, or the grandest expression of the respect we owe to life. It is a wrong belief.

How did that belief come about? I offer a guess. For whatever mischievous historical reason, the ideas of *scientific progress* and the *sanctity of life* have come to hold each other in mutual captivity, and to the mutual detriment of both. For its part, by treating all the causes of death as avoidable evils, equivalent as evils to death itself, medical science has held out the hope that the causes might be eliminated—and has made the promotion of that hope a moral imperative. For its part, a capacious notion of the sanctity of life is ready to play along with scientific ambition: if life is sacred, and death an evil, then it becomes our common duty to support whatever will reduce or eliminate death and enhance life.

A failure to support medical care, some seem to hold, is no less a failure toward the value of life than a failure to enforce laws against murder; the former are just more subtle, discreet, ways of killing people. As Mary Lasker, the celebrated lay lobbyist for the National Institutes of Health in the 1950s and 1960s, once put it, "I'm really opposed to heart attacks and cancer and strokes the way I'm opposed to sin."[13]

What has been the result? Hardly noticing what we were doing, we superimposed upon efforts to control disease and death a structure of moral obligation almost identical to that used earlier in history to judge human actions in the control of voluntary violence and homicide. Our cultural traditions came to give disease, the cause of death, the same status of evildoer as the deliberate human murderer. We cannot put disease in jail, but we can personify it as evil, and we can condemn as hardly less than murderers those who refuse to bring full force of medical science against it. Thus we confused human responsibility in confronting natural evils with that same responsibility in the face of deliberately harmful human actions. We thereby laid upon ourselves an excessive weight of moral obligation, daily visible in the hesitation and often guilt felt by both doctors and families in terminating treatment with the critically ill and dying.

We have thought, by throwing money and research at death, to honor life. But life was of value before modern medicine came to improve upon it. Increased life expectancy was a benefit to human beings, but not because that added *value* to the worth of life. I do not believe that either the most central religious or nonreligious traditions of the sanctity of life hold life as such to be the ultimate value. The latter view, often termed "vitalism," has few avowed defenders. The religious perspectives hold only God to be of ultimate value, whereas most nonreligious traditions would temper a respect for life with a concern for the human capacities of life, which are the source of its value. I will, in any case, mean by the "sanctity of life" the principle that human life is a profoundly high and important value, but not an absolute or unqualified, supreme value.

Yet, somehow, that principle has become distorted and misused. This could not have happened had not the principle come under the sway of the promise of medical power and progress. That promise made it seem plausible for the presumed corollary of the respect for life, the judgment that death is an evil, to have a feasible end point, its elimination by science. Thus was created the perfect double-bind: If you are serious about the value of life and the evil of death, you must not stand in the way of medical science, our best hope to eliminate it. If you hesitate to use that science to its fullest, to give it every benefit of doubt, you are convicted not only of failure of hope for the efficacy of science, but also of a lack of seriousness about the sanctity of life.

This way of thinking might not have taken hold except for

another development. The personification of disease as the evil agent of death has confused and corrupted our understanding of medicine and its relationship to nature. Just as an imputation of universal human responsibility for death has confused our judgment about the appropriate scope of our moral obligation to fight death, so too has the casting of medicine as the sworn enemy of death and disease made a muddle of its role and self-understanding. How has this happened? By taking into itself the principle of the sanctity of life as its unique responsibility and seeing itself as the *only* efficacious agent for promotion of this principle against the ravages of nature, medicine has given itself a holy role, and one sanctioned by society. If the penal system is our agent against the murder and mayhem that human beings wreak upon one another, medicine is our appointed agent against the carnage and destruction wreaked upon us by our biological nature.

In its sanctioned role as the enemy of disease and death, medicine in addition admits of no limits to its aspirations: every disease that can be cured should be cured, and there are none that in principle cannot be cured. Every death that can be averted should be averted, and there are none that in principle cannot be averted. Just as one murder is one too many for a civilized society, so one death from disease is one too many for a decent health-care system.

In the interpretation I am advancing here of the bondage between scientific medicine and the sanctity of life, it is important to understand that this bondage is perfectly compatible with the clinical practice of actually terminating treatment. It is possible to concede that, as matters now stand, a life that is no more than a prolongation of death, a vale of pain, suffering, and decline, need not be vigorously treated. I am here, on the contrary, trying to call attention to the *ideal* of medicine, an ideal that must on occasion be compromised by reality. Disease and death are the ultimate evils, and their eradication the ideal and logical goal of scientific medicine. If, in individual cases, that ideal cannot be achieved, only then it is legitimate to cease trying to struggle against them.

But if that is the case, we can see once again why, for many clinicians and families, death is taken to be a failure, and the need to stop treatment a second-best, lesser-evil choice. The power of this trap is made forcibly apparent when we notice how technological possibility makes increasingly uncertain the line between living and dying, and how at least some medical treatment can be found that will make at least some difference in almost every terminal illness. In that case, the termination of treatment is all too easily construed as an act of omission causing death, and the responsibility for death as the fault, not of nature and disease, but of those who made the choice to terminate.

What am I trying to get at here? My aim is to sever almost entirely the relationship between the technological possibilities of medicine in saving and preserving life, and the value that we should attribute to life. I say "almost" because there is no doubt that medical knowledge and progress can do honor to human life, improving and enhancing it. The error comes in thinking that in medicine the perfect ally has been found to magnify the value of life. That is wrong. The value of life resides in life itself, not in its possibility of being enhanced by medicine. Medicine can improve the *quality* of life, not its value. By exactly the same reasoning, medicine can also be seen as posing hazards to the quality of life, but not to the value of life. The mistake is to think that medical knowledge invariably enhances life and is thus the natural savior of the sanctity of life. It is by no means automatic and inevitable that medicine will enhance life; it may or may not, depending on how it is deployed. Yet the belief in medicine and a commitment to respect life have been allowed to reinforce each other mutually in dangerous and muddlesome ways.

Why Is It So Hard to Die a Peaceful Death?

In the previous chapter, I raised the question: why is it so difficult to die a tame or peaceful death? The two reasons I offered were the increasing difficulty of finding any clear line between living and dying, a result of technological advances; and the ambivalence, exacerbated by medical science, that many feel about whether death should be fought or accepted. In this chapter, I have added three more reasons why it is so hard to die a peaceful death.

The first is that medical science has averted its eyes almost altogether from the biological fact of mortality, unchanged for the human species, and focused its attention single-mindedly on the causes of death. This focus has had some unhappy consequences, most notably fostering the illusion that mortality can be eliminated by eradicating lethal disease—an illusion that has led to a medicine beset by excessive pressure to combat the causes of death, and the belief, therefore, that death from disease is intolerable. A second reason stems from the widespread belief, deeply embedded in medicine and public life, that the old-time powers of nature have been replaced by human agency. Death is no longer the fault of nature; it has become an exclusively human responsibility. The practical consequence of this development is to make it more difficult to terminate treatment, now taken to carry as much moral weight and responsibility as direct killing. The third reason is that, in the conflation of respect for the sanctity of life and the technological imperative, medicine and morality have combined to create a powerful pressure against acceptance of death. Both science, with its own imperative, and ethics, with one no less potent, have joined forces to declare death the enemy. To accept death, many seem to think, is to reject both modern medicine and the value of human life, an unacceptable rejection of new and old values.

If any one of these reasons is in itself sufficient to make a peaceful death more difficult, their combined force is positively ferocious. They have created harmful pressures on medicine to distort its own nature by subordinating its full mission to the combating of death. They have put needless and confusing burdens on human choice by giving those choices an omnipotence, a power once reserved to God, that of being responsible for all of nature. They have no less put a false and impossible burden on morality, making any effort to stand in the way of the eradication of death an offense against both science and morality, an onus few are willing to bear.

We can now, I think, see the full dimensions of the "wild death" identified by Philippe Ariès. It is wild not simply because it is out of control and terrorizing in its modern incarnation, but also because, in the name of combating mortality, it has managed simultaneously to subvert the institution of medicine, which cannot overcome mortality, and the morality of human decisions about life and death, which should not have to bear the burden of omni-responsibility.

In the rise of interest in euthanasia and assisted suicide, we can see the last act of this drama being played out, and to that I will now turn.

Chapter 3

THE LAST ILLUSION:
REGULATING EUTHANASIA

The figure of death as a stalker, lying in wait for us, is old and familiar. In earlier times, it sought people throughout life, but was more likely to catch them in childhood than in their old age. We have in our day learned increasingly well how to push death from the young to the old. If it still relentlessly pursues us, we have found that we can also pursue it. We do so by trying to live healthier lives and by making use of medical knowledge to catch death in its lair, to do unto it what it would do unto us.

In the end, that effort fails. It is a one-sided struggle. Death can kill us, but we cannot kill death. We can only hold it off for a time. Yet there is also something else we can try to do: to see if it is possible to die in a way we find peaceful and tolerable. It is a mistake, however, to think that we can, simultaneously, pursue a maximal technological effort to sustain life and still hope for a peaceful death. Technology cannot be managed with that kind of dominance and delicacy. Despite the understandable enthusiasm for advance directives, those efforts have, for the most part, fallen short, and are likely to continue doing so as a means to gain control of our dying. For all of their value in allowing us to express our wishes, they have not greatly succeeded either in reducing the anxiety of those fearful of death at the hands of modern medicine or in cutting through the deep complexities of terminating treatment in the face of technological medicine.' "Good death" "mercy killing" "Physician Assisted Suicide"

The euthanasia movement represents a powerful effort to move beyond that impasse, to take the last, definitive, step in gaining full individual self-determination. It seeks to reassure us we can die as we choose, and to provide a technically decisive solution to our dying. However mistaken in its direction and emphasis— as I will argue it is—a turn to euthanasia is a perfectly understandable, not unreasonable, response to a death that is increasingly difficult to make peaceful, that is ever more ensnared in technological and moral traps. On the one hand, there are all the obstacles thrown in the way of simply allowing people to die from disease: medicine's conflation of the value of the sanctity of life and the technological imperative, rendering an acceptance of death morally suspect. On the other hand, because all deaths are increasingly judged to be a human responsibility, with the distinction between omission and commission erased, there is now every incentive to seek a final and decisive control over the process of dying. Euthanasia and assisted suicide present, seemingly, the perfect way to do just that.

The euthanasia movement rests on two basic claims, secondarily supported by other considerations as well. Those claims are our right to self-determination, and the obligation we owe to one another to relieve suffering, but especially the obligation of the physician to do so. Its deepest point might simply be understood as this: if we cannot trust disease to take our lives quickly or peacefully, nor can we rely on doctors to know with great precision how or when to stop treatment to allow that to happen, then we have a right to turn to more direct means. Physicians should be allowed, in the name of mercy, to end our lives at our voluntary request or, alternatively, permitted to put into our hands the means that will allow us to commit suicide. We will then be assured a peaceful death, one that we have fashioned for ourselves. In place of the tame death no longer (if ever assuredly and perfectly) given us by nature, we must shape, by our choice, one of our own making.

This is a dangerous direction to go in the search for a peaceful death. It rests on the illusion that a society can safely put in the private hands of physicians the power directly and deliberately to take life. It threatens to add to an already sorry human history of giving one person the liberty to take the life of another still a further sad chapter. It perpetuates and pushes to an extreme the very ideology of control, the goal of mastering life and death, that created the problems of modern medicine in the first place. Instead of changing the medicine generating the problem of an intolerable death, it simply treats the symptoms, all the while reinforcing, and driving us more deeply into, an ideology of control.

I will reserve for the next chapter an alternative to that ideology, and will examine here the arguments advanced in favor of euthanasia. Those arguments are forceful and appealing. They also have a special attraction, sometimes overlooked: they take some commonly accepted values, by no means radical, and push them along one step further. The deepest of these values is that human beings have a right to manage their own destinies in the face of natural evils. The British Earl of Listowel articulates that value in a familiar way when he writes that "social progress can be measured by the degree of control man achieves over his environment by substituting his rational will for the blind and instinctive forces of nature. In the cycle of human life we have gone far toward mastering the processes of reproduction. But the process of dying is still left mainly to chance and the disintegration of the body."[1]

The fear of dying is powerful. Even more powerful sometimes is the fear of *not* dying, of being a burden on one's family, of being forced to endure destructive pain or to live out a life of unrelieved, pointless suffering. The provocations to embrace euthanasia can seem compelling: prolonged agony, a sense of utter futility, pain that can only be relieved at the price of oblivion, a desperate gasping for breath which, if relieved, will be followed again and again by the same gasping; or, perhaps even worse, months or years in a nursing home. The possibilities of inhuman suffering should not be minimized, and I do not want to rest my resistance on any slighting of that kind. I can well imagine situations that could drive me to want such relief or feel driven to want it for others. It is not easy to say no to something so attractive, so seemingly patent in its possibility to relieve our fear. And public opinion is not saying no. Instead it shows a striking shift toward saying yes.[2] The movement to legalize euthanasia and assisted suicide is a strong and, seemingly, historically inevitable response to the fear I have described. It draws part of its strength from the failure of modern medicine to reassure us that it can manage our dying with dignity and comfort. It draws another part from our desire to be masters of our fate. Why must we endure that which need not be endured? If medicine cannot always bring us the kind of death we might like through its technical skills, why can it not use these skills to give us a quick and merciful release?

The Relief of Suffering: Virtues and Duties

No moral impulse seems more deeply embedded than the need to relieve human suffering. It is a basic tenet of the great religions of the world. It has become a foundation stone for the practice of medicine, and it is at the core of the social and welfare programs of all civilized nations. Unless we have been brutalized, our feelings numbed by cruelty or systematic indifference, we cannot stand to see another person suffer. The tears of another, even a total stranger, can bring tears to our own eyes. At the heart of the virtue of compassion is the capacity to feel with, and for, another. In those closest to us, that virtue often leads us to feel the pain of another as if it were our own. And sometimes it is stronger than that: it is a source of intensified anguish that we cannot lift from another the pain we would, if we could, make our own. A parent feels that way about the suffering of a child, and a spouse or a friend about the suffering of a loved one who is trapped by pain.

Yet for all the depth of our common response to suffering, our general agreement as a civilized society that it should be relieved, the scope and depth of that moral duty is not clear, especially for physicians. The problem of euthanasia forces us to answer a hard question: ought the general duty of the physician to relieve suffering encompass the right to kill a patient if, in the judgment of the patient, that is desired and seems necessary? The question can be put from the patient's viewpoint as well: is it a legitimate moral request for a patient to ask her doctor to kill her, or assist her to commit suicide?

Some initial clarifications are necessary. It is part of our common speech to refer to the relief of "pain and suffering," as if they were identical. Yet as Dr. Eric Cassell has reminded us, they are not the same, even if there can be considerable overlap. Pain ordinarily refers to a highly distressful, undesirable sensation or experience ordinarily associated with a physical cause.[3] A precise definition is, however, elusive. There are many forms of pain—"burning," "stabbing," "gnawing" are only some of the many terms used to describe different experiences of pain—and there are also many different possible meanings to be attributed to the pain. Pain cannot be well understood apart from those meanings, which influence the effect of the pain upon the person, not just the person's body.[4] Suffering, by contrast, ordinarily refers to a person's psychological or spiritual state, and is characteristically marked by a sense of anguish, dread, foreboding, futility, meaninglessness, or a range of other emotions associated with a loss of meaning or control or both. Not all pain leads to suffering (the pain of the victorious distance runner leads to pleasure), nor does suffering require the presence of physical pain (the anguish of knowing one has Alzheimer's disease). Chronic, unrelieved pain is likely to be a source of suffering, but the meaning attributed to the pain will make a great difference in how oppressive the pain is taken to be. The greatest sense of suffering is likely to come when pain, or a deadly illness, seems to threaten the integrity and intactness of one's personhood, threatening it with disintegration, a loss of a sense of an ordered, integrated self.[5]

What should be done in response to such suffering? Is it simply a *nice* thing to relieve suffering if we can, a gesture of charity or kindness worthy of praise?[6] We might say that it is good to cultivate and express our impulse of compassion, that we will all be better off if we entertain that as an ideal in our lives together. Or is there more to it? Might it be that the relief of suffering is a moral *duty*, not just a noble ideal, to which we are obliged even if our sense of compassion is faint, even if what is asked of us might cause some suffering on our own part? How far and in what way, that is, does our duty extend in the relief of suffering, and just what kind of suffering is encompassed within such a duty?

One common answer to questions of that kind is that we are, at the least, obliged to relieve the suffering of others when we can do so at no high cost to ourselves, and we should do so when the suffering at stake is unnecessary. But that does not tell us much that is helpful, though it is surely important to repeatedly remind ourselves and others of such obligations. The hard cases are those where the demands upon us may be morally or psychologically stressful, and where there is uncertainty about the significance of the suffering.

There are two burdens that it is useful to distinguish. One of them is where the demand upon us is to act, to do something specifically to relieve the suffering. That may mean giving our already overcrowded time just to be with someone in pain, whose need is for companionship, for closeness; or perhaps providing needed money to improve the nursing care of a dying parent; or taking the trouble to find a better doctor, or hospital, for a spouse receiving poor care. Demands of that kind can be heavy, pressing our sense of duty to the limit, and sometimes it can be unclear just where the limit is.

The other burden is more subtle, that of knowing when suffering cannot, or should not, be wholly overcome, and where our duty may be accepting the suffering of another, just as the person whose suffering it is must accept it. Many legitimate moral demands, for instance, will carry with them the possibility of suffering, and they should not for that reason be shirked. To take an unpopular position, to stand up for one's rights, to remain true to one's promises and commitments can all entail unavoidable suffering. A parent's commitment to the good of a child may require, and probably will at times require, that for the sake of the child's development the parent accept the child's need to bear the penalties of its own choices and mistakes, and thereby to suffer. The same can be said of many other human relationships—friends and lovers, husbands and wives. As bystanders to the suffering, we have to accept its unavoidability for the sufferer. We cannot relieve that suffering. The demand in some cases is to accept the suffering that another must endure, not run from it. Patience, loyalty, steadfastness, fortitude are called for in dealing with the person who must suffer, to help and allow the person to do and be what he must, however heavy the burden on him and others. We are called upon to suffer with the other, to be a supportive presence.

For just those reasons it cannot be fully correct to say that our highest moral duty to one another is the relief of suffering. More precisely, our duty is to enhance the good and the welfare of one another. The relief of suffering will ordinarily be an important way to accomplish that, but not always. What we need to know is whether the suffering exists because without it some other human good cannot be accomplished; and that is exactly the case with the suffering caused by living out one's moral duties or ideals for a life.

Therein lies the ambiguity of the term "unnecessary suffering," frequently invoked as the kind of suffering euthanasia can obviate. Suffering will surely be "unnecessary" when it serves no purpose, when it is not an inextricable part of achieving important human goals. Unavoidable necessary suffering, by contrast, is that which is the essential means, or accompaniment, of valuable human ends; and not all suffering is. Yet the real problem here is in deciding upon our goals, and the hardest choice will be in deciding whether, and how, to pursue goals that may entail suffering. If we make the relief of suffering itself the highest goal, we run the severe risk of sacrificing, or minimizing, other human purposes. Life would then be focused on avoiding pain, minimizing risk, and craftily eyeing all possible life projects and goals with a view toward their likelihood of producing suffering.

If that is hardly desirable in the living of our individual lives, it is no less problematic in devising social policy. A society ought, so far as it can, to work for the relief of pain and suffering; that is to state a simple moral principle. But a more complex principle is needed: a society should work to relieve only that suffering which is not an unavoidable part of living out its other values and aspirations. That means it must ask, on the one hand, what those values are or should be, and, on the other, what policies for the relief of suffering might subvert its general values.

The most profound question we must then ask is this: if the suffering of illness and death come from the deep assault on our sense of integrity and self-direction, what is the best way we can—as those who give care, who want to do right by a person— honor that integrity? The claim of euthanasia proponents is that the assault of terminal illness upon the self is legitimately relieved, even mercifully and honorably so, by recognizing the right to self-determination, and that what the individual wants—a deliberately chosen death administered (or assisted) by another— is appropriate as a way of relieving suffering. Yet notice what we have accepted here. It is the idea that our integrity can *only* be served by the self-determination that brings death, by the direct implication of another in our death, and by the acceptance of the implicit assumption that the suffering is "unnecessary"— meaningless, avoidable. To accept that comes close to declaring that life can only have meaning if marked by self-determination, a strange notion indeed, flying directly in the face of human experience. That experience shows that a noble and heroic life

" STRAW MAN"

can be achieved by those who have little or no control over the external conditions of their lives, but have the wisdom and dignity necessary to fashion a meaningful life without it.

We would also be declaring that a life not marked by self-control, self-determination, is a meaningless one once burdened with unwanted suffering. It is not for nothing perhaps that modern medicine, in its quest for cure, has, as Stanley Hauerwas has reminded us, itself contributed to the idea that all suffering is pointless, representing not life and its natural condition but the failure of medicine to overcome, or relieve, that condition.[7]

But might it not be said, in response, that granting social permission for euthanasia would not be taking a general position at all on the meaning of life, death, and suffering, but only empowering each individual and his or her accomplice physician to make that determination themselves? Would it not be, in that sense, socially neutral? Not at all. To establish euthanasia as social policy is, first, to side with those who say that some suffering is meaningless and unnecessary, to be relieved as decisively as possible, and that only individuals can determine what such suffering that is; and, second, to say that such a highly variable, highly subjective matter is best left to the irrevocable judgment of doctor and patient. That is not a neutral policy at all, but one that makes a decisive judgment about what constitutes an appropriate, socially acceptable response to dying, the mutually agreed-upon killing of a person; and about social policy, the legitimation of direct killing as a response to perceived threats of suffering and loss of self-integrity.

A great hazard of this approach is that it declares some forms of human suffering—but only those forms determined by private, variable responses—to be beyond human help and caring, open only to death as a solution. Dr. Timothy E. Quill, justifying his assistance to his patient Diane in her decision to commit suicide, said he was afraid that "the preoccupation with her fear of a lingering death would interfere with Diane's getting the most out of the time she had left until she found a safe way to ensure her death."[8] He made clear that he was treating her desire for control and for a certain kind of life as much as her medical needs. He became a doctor of her soul, so to speak, not just of her body. Yet why should he have accepted her "preoccupation" or her longing for control as either decisive or unalterable, much less as a problem that it was appropriate for him as a *doctor* to address, her particular way of wanting to live and to value a life? Simply because a patient so declares her values? It is a striking break with both the medical and moral traditions of medicine to treat the desires and wishes of patients as if they alone provide legitimation of a doctor's skills. That stance is to make doctors artisans in the fashioning of a patient's life—and in this case death—a role well beyond the traditional and reasonable range of medicine, that of restoring or maintaining health.

There is little disagreement about the duty of the physician to relieve physical pain, even though there are some significant disputes about how far that effort should go. Of more pertinence to my concern here, however, is the extent of the duty of the physician to relieve suffering—that is, to try to relieve the psychological or spiritual condition of a person who, as a result of illness, suffers (whether in pain or not). I want to contend that the duty is important, but limited.

Two Levels of Suffering

Two levels of suffering can be distinguished. At one level, the principal problem is that of the fear, uncertainty, dread, or anguish of the sick person in coping with the illness and its meaning for the continuation of life and intact personhood—what might be called the psychological penumbra of illness. At a second level, the problem touches on the meaning of suffering for the meaning of life itself. The question here is more fundamental: what does my suffering tell me about the point or purpose or end of human existence, most notably my own? The questions here no longer are just psychological but encompass fundamental philosophical and religious questions.

The physician should do all in his or her power to respond, as a physician, to the first level, but it is inappropriate, I contend, to attempt to solve by lethal means the problems that arise at the second level. What would that distinction mean in practice? It means that the doctor should, through counseling, pain relief, and cooperative efforts with family and friends, do everything possible to reduce the sense of dread and anxiety, of disintegration of self, in the face of a threatened death. The doctor should provide care, comfort, and compassion. But when the patient says to the doctor that life no longer has meaning, or that the suffering cannot be borne because of its perceived pointlessness, or that a loss of control is experienced as an intolerable insult to a patient's sense of dignity—at that point, the doctor must draw a line. Those problems cannot properly be solved by medicine, and it is a mistake for medicine even to make an attempt to do so.

The purpose of medicine is not to relieve all the problems of human mortality, the most central and difficult of which is why we have to die at all or die in ways that seem pointless to us. It is not the purpose of medicine to give us control over our human destiny, or to help us devise a life to our private specifications— and especially the specification most desired these days, that of complete control over death and its circumstances. That is not the role of medicine, because it has no competence to manage the meaning of life and death—the deepest and oldest human questions—but only some of the physical and psychological manifestations of those problems.

Medicine's role must be limited to what it can do, which is to relieve pain, and to bring comfort to those who suffer psychologically because of illness. That is all, and that is enough. When the physician would use medical knowledge, designed to help with that task, to cause death directly as a way of solving a patient's problems with life and mortality itself, he goes too far, exceeding his own professional and moral rights and those of the profession to which he belongs. There has been a longstanding, historical resistance to giving physicians the power to kill, precisely because of the skill they could bring to that task: if their technical power to kill were matched by a moral or legal authority to kill or assist in suicide, the way would be open for a corruption of their vocation.

I do not claim that a sharp and precise line can always be found between the two levels, but only that some limits can be feasibly set to enable us to say when the physician has strayed too far into the thickets of the second level. For ordinary purposes, it remains appropriate to speak about the duty of the physician to "relieve pain and suffering," but only as long as it is understood that this can be done only to relieve the problems of illness, not the problems of life itself. What life itself may give us at its end is a death that seems, in the suffering it brings, to make no sense. That is a *terrible* problem, but it is the patient's problem, not the doctor's. The doctor can relieve pain if it is present, make the patient as comfortable as possible, and be another human presence. Otherwise, the patient must be on his or her own. We have no resource left but ourselves at that point.

There is also another side to the issue. When euthanasia is requested, the doctor is being asked to act upon someone else's subjective suffering—variable from person to person, externally unverifiable, and always, in principle, reversible—but to respond with an action that will be objective and irreversible. As the human response to evil and suffering suggest, there is nothing in a particular burden on human life, or in the nature of suffering itself, that *necessarily* and *inevitably* leads to a desire to be dead, much less a will to bring death about. That will and must always be a function of the patient's values and the way they are either legitimated or rejected by the culture of which that patient is a part. Suffering in and of itself is not a good clinical predictor of a desire to be dead; depression is a far better predictor of a desire for suicide than illness, pain, or old age.[9] If that is the case, then we have a complex, double challenge before us: to determine whether, under those ambiguous circumstances, we should empower one person to kill another; and, if so, what the moral standard should be for the one who is to do the killing.

Self-Determination and Private Killing

Perhaps the most compelling attraction of euthanasia is that it appears to be simply one more logical, much overdue, extension of a right long recognized in this country. Just over a century ago, in the 1891 *Union Pacific* v. *Botsford* case, the Supreme Court held: "No right is more sacred, or is more carefully guarded, by the common law, than the right of the individual to the possession and control of his own person."[10] That right has been reaffirmed time and again, and especially underscored in those rulings—most recently the Nancy Cruzan case—that declare our right to terminate medical treatment and thus to die.

But if it should happen to be impossible for us to bring about our own death so easily, would it not be reasonable to ask someone else, specifically a doctor, to help us die? Would it not, moreover, be an act of mercy for a doctor to give us such a release? Is not the relief of suffering a high moral good? To say no in response to questions of that kind seems both repressive and cruel. They invoke our cherished political values of liberty and self-determination. They draw upon our deep and long-standing moral commitment to the relief of suffering. They bespeak our ancient efforts to triumph over death, to find a way to bring it to heel.

Nonetheless, we should as a society reject, and decisively so, euthanasia and assisted suicide. If a death marked by pain or suffering is a nasty death, a natural biological evil of a supreme kind, euthanasia and assisted suicide are wrong and harmful responses to that evil. To kill another person directly—in the name of mercy and that person's self-determination (as I will define "euthanasia" here)—or to assist another to commit suicide (logically little different from euthanasia) would add still another to a society already burdened with man-made evils.[11]

Euthanasia is mistakenly understood as only a personal matter of self-determination, the control of our own bodies, just a small step beyond our already available legal right to commit suicide. But, unlike suicide, an act carried out by the person herself, euthanasia should be understood as of its nature a social act. It requires the assistance of someone else and could not take place without it. Legalizing euthanasia would also provide an important social sanction for the practice, tacitly legitimating it, and affecting many aspects of our society beyond the immediate relief of suffering individuals. It would change the traditional role of the physician. It would require the regulation and oversight of government. It would add to the acceptable range of permissible killing in our society one more occasion for the taking of life.

We might decide we are as a people prepared to live with those implications. But we should not deceive ourselves: euthanasia and assisted suicide represent a radical move into an entirely different realm of morality, that of the killing of one person by another.

All civilized societies have developed laws to reduce the occasions on which one person is allowed to kill another. All have resisted the notion that private agreements can be reached allowing one person to take the life of another to serve the interests of one or both parties. Traditionally, three circumstances only have made the taking of a life acceptable: killing in self-defense or to protect another life, in the course of a just war, and in capital punishment. Killing both in war and by capital punishment have been opposed by some; capital punishment is now banned in many countries, most notably in Western Europe.

Apart from those long-standing debates, what is most striking about the historically licit conditions of killing is the requirement: (1) that killing is only permissible when relatively objective standards have been met—a genuine threat to life or vital goods in the case of killing in self-defense and warfare, the absence of an alternative means of meeting those threats, and a strict limit on the killing; and (2) that the public and not solely a private good is thereby served. In the case of self-defense, the permission to kill helps foster a sense of public security in the face of personal threats, for instance.

The proposal to legalize active euthanasia and assisted suicide is nothing less than a proposal to add a new category of acceptable killing to those already socially legitimated. To do so would be to reverse the long-developing trend to limit the occasions of legally sactioned killing (most notable in the campaigns to abolish capital punishment and to limit access to handguns). Civilized societies have slowly come to understand how virtually impossible it is to control even legally sanctioned killing. No matter how carefully safeguards are fashioned, abuse and corruption are invited.

Euthanasia would reinstate private killings. By "private killings" I mean those in which the agreement of one person to kill another is ratified in private by the persons themselves, not by public authorities (even if it is made legal and safeguards are put into effect). Do we want to give one person the right to kill another for the sake of the relief of pain and suffering? That is the question before us.

It is noteworthy that the law does not allow, in the United States or elsewhere, the right of one person to kill another even if the latter requests, or consents, that it be done. All civilized societies have also outlawed private killings, either in the name of honor (such as dueling), or to right private wrongs (such as to avenge adulterous relationships). Yet if we generally accept in our society a right to control our own lives and bodies, why has the extension of that right to private killing been denied?

The most obvious reason is a reluctance to give one person absolute and irrevocable power over the life of another, whether there is consent or not. That prohibition is a way of saying that the social stakes in the legitimation of killing are extraordinarily high. It is to recognize that a society should—for the mutual protection of all—be exceedingly sparing in conferring a right to kill on anyone, much less in advancing the personal goals of those to be killed, however understandable or otherwise appealing they may be.

John Stuart Mill, in his classic essay *On Liberty*, noted that civilized societies do not legally permit individuals the right to sell themselves into slavery, even though that denial is a limitation on self-determination. "The principle of freedom," he wrote, "cannot require that he should be free not to be free. It is not freedom to be allowed to alienate his freedom."[12] Yet it is not just the ceding of freedom that is problematic. The absolute power that is put into the hands of another, I would add—the right to be a slaveholder—is not compatible with respect for our human dignity. Both the slaveholder and the enslaved are corrupted by the relationship, even if both have the good of the other as their motive. The one gives up too much, and the other has too much given him.

A similar consideration applies in the case of killings authorized in the name of mercy: they give one person an absolute power over another. Our right to self-determination can be likened, as Joel Feinberg has put it, to an absolute sovereignty. Our lives are our own, not someone else's: "There is no such thing as 'trivial interference' with personal sovereignty; nor is it simply another value to be weighed in cost-benefit comparison. In this respect, if not others, a trivial interference with sovereignty is like a minor invasion of virginity: the logic of each concept is such that a value is respected in its entirety or not at all."[13]

Understood one way, this is exactly the kind of argument that might conventionally be taken to justify euthanasia. I draw exactly the opposite conclusion (though Feinberg does not). We cannot, I believe, transfer our sovereignty to another without contradicting it. A sovereignty that can legally and morally be given away is fragile and contingent, not sovereignty at all. To allow another person to kill us is the most radically imaginable relinquishment of sovereignty, not just one more way of exercising it. Our life belongs no longer to us, but to the person into whose power we give it. No person should have that kind of power over another, freely gained or not. No defender of civil liberties and the right of self-determination should want to see that possibility available.

Does it not make a difference that the absolute power is given, not to subjugate another (as in slavery), but as an act of mercy, to bring relief from suffering? No. Although the motive may be more benign than in the case of slavery as usually understood, that motive is beside the point. The aim in prohibiting euthanasia is to avoid introducing into society the inherent corruption of legitimated private killing. "All power corrupts," Lord Acton wrote, "and absolute power corrupts absolutely." It is that profound insight—a reflection on human despotism, usually justified initially out of good, empathetic motives—that should be kept in mind when we would give one person the right to kill another.

The Boundless Logic of Private Killing

We come here to a striking pitfall of the common argument for euthanasia and assisted suicide. Once the key premises of that argument are accepted, there will remain no logical way in the future to: (1) deny euthanasia to anyone who requests it for whatever reason, terminal illness or not; or to (2) deny it to the suffering incompetent, even if they do not request it. We can erect legal safeguards and specify required procedures to keep these things from happening. But over time the safeguards will provide poor protection if the logic of the moral premises upon which they are based are fatally flawed. They will appear arbitrary and flimsy, and will invite covert evasion or outright rejection.

Where are the flaws here? Recall that there are two classical arguments in favor of euthanasia and assisted suicide: our right of self-determination, and our claim upon the mercy of others, especially doctors, to relieve our suffering if they can do so.[14] These two arguments are typically spliced together and presented as a single contention. Yet if they are considered independently—and there is no inherent reason why they must be linked—they display serious problems. Consider, first, the argument for our right of self-determination. It is said that a competent adult person ought to have a right to euthanasia for the relief of suffering. But why must the person be suffering? Does not that stipulation already compromise the right of self-determination? How can self-determination have any limits? Why are not the person's desires or motives, whatever they be, sufficient? How can we justify this arbitrary limitation of self-determination? The standard arguments for euthanasia offer no answers to those questions.

Consider next the person who is suffering but not competent, perhaps demented or mentally retarded. The standard argument would deny euthanasia to that person. But why? It would seem grossly unfair to deny such a person relief simply because he lacked competence. Are the incompetent less entitled to relief from suffering than the competent? Will it only be affluent middle-class people, mentally fit and able, who can qualify? Will those who are incompetent but suffering be denied what those who are intellectually and emotionally better off can have? Would that be fair? Do they suffer less for being incompetent? The standard argument about our duty to relieve suffering offers no response to those questions either.

Is it, however, fair to euthanasia advocates to do what I have done, to separate, and treat individually, the two customary arguments in favor of a legal right to euthanasia? The implicit reason for joining them is no doubt the desire to avoid abuse. The aim of requiring a demonstration of suffering and terminal illness is to exclude perfectly healthy people from demanding that, in the name of self-determination and for their own private reasons, another person be called upon to kill them. The aim of requiring a show of mental competence to effect self-determination is to exclude the nonvoluntary or involuntary killing of the depressed, the retarded, and the demented.

My contention is that the joining of those two requirements is perfectly arbitrary, a jerry-rigged combination if ever there was one. Each has its own logic, and each could be used to justify euthanasia. But, in the nature of the case, that logic, it seems evident, offers little resistance to denying any competent person the right to be killed, sick or not; and little resistance to killing the incompetent, as long as there is good reason to believe they are suffering. There is no principled reason to reject such logic, and no reason to think it could long remain suppressed by the expedient of an arbitrary legal stipulation that both features, suffering and competence, be present.

One related problem is worth considering. If the act of euthanasia, conventionally understood, requires the request and consent of the patient, it requires no less that the person who is to do the killing have his or her own independent moral standards for acceding to the request. The doctor must act with integrity. How can a doctor who voluntarily brings about, or is instrumental in, the death of another legitimately justify that to himself? Would the mere claim of self-determination on the part of someone be sufficient: "It is my body, doctor, and I request that you kill me"? There is a historical resistance to that kind of claim, and doctors quite rightly have never been willing to do what patients want solely because they want it. This would reduce the doctors' role to that of an automaton, subordinating their integrity to patients' wishes or demands. There is surely a legitimate fear, moreover, that, if such claim were sanctioned, there would be no reason to forbid any two competent persons from entering into an agreement for one to kill the other, a form of consenting-adult killing. Perhaps it also arises out of a reluctance to put doctors in the position of taking life simply as a means of advancing patient self-determination, quite apart from any medical reasons for doing so.

Yet the most likely reason for resistance to a pure self-determination standard is that our culture has, traditionally, defined the appropriate role of the physician as someone whose duty it is to promote and restore health. It has thus been customary, even among those pressing for euthanasia, to hang on to some part of the physician's traditional role. That is why a mere claim of self-determination, requiring no reference to health at all, is not enough. A doctor will not cut off my healthy arm simply because I decide my autonomy and well-being would thereby be enhanced.

What may we conclude from these still-viable traditions? For a doctor to justify committing an act of euthanasia, he must have his own independent moral standards to maintain his integrity.

What should those standards be? The doctor will not be able to use a *medical* standard. A euthanasia decision is not a medical but a moral decision. The doctor must believe that a life of subjectively experienced intense suffering is not worth living if she is to be justified in taking the decisive and ultimate step of killing the patient. It must be *her* moral reason to act, not the patient's reason (even though they may coincide). But if she believes that a life of some forms of suffering is not worth living, then how can she deny the same relief to a person who cannot request it, or who requests it but whose competence is in doubt? There is no self-evident reason why the supposed duty to relieve suffering must be limited to competent patients claiming self-determination. Or why patients who claim death as their right under self-determination must be either suffering or dying.

There is, moreover, the possibility that what begins as a right of doctors to kill under specified conditions will soon become a duty to kill. On what grounds could a doctor deny a request by a competent person for euthanasia? It is not sufficient just to stipulate that no doctor be required to do that which violates his conscience. As commonly articulated, the argument about why a doctor has a right to perform euthanasia—the dual duty to respect patient self-determination and to relieve suffering—is said to be central to the vocation of being a doctor. Why should duties as weighty as those be set aside on the grounds of "conscience" or "personal values"?

Such puzzles make clear that the moral situation is radically changed once our self-determination requires the participation and assistance of a doctor. It is no longer a solitary act, but a two-person, social, act. That doctor's moral life and integrity are also, and no less, encompassed in the act of euthanasia. What, we might then ask, should be the appropriate moral standards for a person asked to kill another? What are the appropriate virtues and sensitivities of such a person? How should that person think of his or her own life and find, within that life, a place for the killing of another person? The language of a presumed right of someone to kill another to relieve suffering obscures questions of that kind.

Now, I could imagine someone granting the weight of the considerations against euthanasia I have advanced and yet having this response: "Is not our duty to relieve suffering sufficiently strong to justify running some risks? Why should we be intimidated by the dangers in a decisive relief of suffering? Is not the present situation, where death can be slow, painful, and full of suffering, already a clear and present danger?"

Our duty to relieve suffering—by no means unlimited, in any case—cannot justify the introduction of new evils into society. The risk of doing just that in the legalization of euthanasia is too great, particularly since the number of people whose pain and suffering could not be otherwise relieved would never be large (as even most euthanasia advocates recognize). It is too great because it would take a disproportionate social change to bring it about, one whose implications extend far beyond the sick and dying, reaching into the practice of medicine and into the sphere of socially sanctioned killing. It is too great because, as the history of the twentieth century should demonstrate, killing is a contagious disease, not easy to stop once unleashed in society. It is too great because it would offer medicine too convenient a way out of its hardest cases, those where there is ample room for further, more benign, reforms. We are far from exhausting the known remedies for the relief of pain (frequently, even routinely, underused), and a long way from providing decent psychological support for those who, not necessarily in pain, nonetheless suffer because of despair and a sense of futility in continuing life.

The legalization of euthanasia is, finally, too great a risk because it would lend credence to the mistaken notion that a self-chosen death is a "rational" way to deal with suffering. It is probably no coincidence that the Romans, who justified suicide on the grounds that our bodies are a form of property, also justified slavery on similar grounds, that one person may own the body of another. The great philosopher Immanuel Kant argued that "to use the power of free will for its own destruction is self-contradictory. If freedom is the condition of life it cannot be employed to abolish life and so to destroy and abolish itself. To use life for its own destruction, to use life for producing lifelessness, is self-contradictory."[15] I will not pursue here the question of suicide, but only repeat that, in addition to the powerful case made by Kant against suicide, the only solid *predictor* of suicide is a history of depression. Otherwise, suicide follows no *rational pattern* in its manifestation, a necessary condition if one is to speak of "rational" suicide.

Physical pain and psychological suffering in the critically ill and dying are great evils. The attempt to relieve them by the introduction of euthanasia and assisted suicide is an even greater evil. Those practices threaten the future security of the living. They no less threaten the dying themselves. Once a society allows one person to take the life of another based on their mutual private standards of a life worth living, there can be no safe or sure way to contain the deadly virus thus introduced. It will go where it will thereafter.

The Dutch Experience

The Dutch experience with euthanasia, now practiced in that country for over a decade, provides a pertinent example of just how it is likely to happen. The similarity between the moral and political values of the Netherlands and those of the United States makes that case all the more pointed in its significance. Euthanasia and assisted suicide are technically still illegal in Holland. During the late 1970s and early 1980s, however, the Dutch courts declared in a number of decisions that euthanasia carried out by physicians would not be prosecuted if three conditions were met.[16] First, the person requesting euthanasia must be a competent adult, and his or her request one that has been persistently made over time. Second, the patient must be in a state of "unbearable" pain or suffering. Third, the independent judg-ment of a second doctor must be obtained to verify the first two conditions. In addition to these three requirements, existing laws require that there be accurate reporting by the physician of the cause of death.

What has been the result? Some recent Dutch studies, in-cluding one commissioned by the government, provide some illuminating information. The best estimates are that there are between twenty-three hundred and four thousand cases a year.[17] A large portion are thought to take place at home rather than in hospitals. There are some reasons to be disturbed by the Dutch experience. Despite the large number of estimated cases each year, not more than three hundred are actually reported, as the law requires. This means that there is *no way at all* of knowing whether the other conditions specified by the Dutch Supreme Court are actually being met. Is there always voluntary consent? Are all the patients competent? Is the suffering thought to be unbearable? Is a second opinion being asked for? No one knows with any certainty. Since the Dutch experience is often adduced as an instance of the way in which a sensible, safe regulation of euthanasia can be implemented, this is a major failing. It means that, in fact, despite the Court's required conditions, there is no effective legal oversight of euthanasia in Holland, and no evi-dence that the Court's conditions are taken seriously. No efforts of any consequence, moreover, are made by the Dutch police authorities to seek out those practicing euthanasia without re-porting it. Unless they act in some flagrant way, doctors who ignore the Court's conditions seem to do so with legal impunity.

Perhaps most disturbing to me in that respect was the appar-ently indifferent response to the situation I encountered among a group of prominent supporters of, and spokespersons for, eu-thanasia during a late-1990 visit to Holland.[18] They conceded that the small number of reported cases did raise some basic doubts about the operation of the Court's standards, but this did not, seemingly, disturb anyone. They agreed that it would be good to have better data on the actual practice, and said that a study was under way—the Remmelink Report—to do just that; but they seemed willing enough to tolerate the present ignorance about whether the required patient safeguards really work. They conceded as well that there probably have been some cases of nonvoluntary euthanasia (with children and demented elderly patients). And the Remmelink Report, determining that there are some 1,000 cases of nonvoluntary (unrequested) cases a year (0.8% of all deaths), later lent statistical support to that admission.

As for the required diagnosis of "unbearable" suffering, it was agreed that this cannot be a purely medical judgment; it depends upon the values of the physician no less than those of the patient. A physician from a Dutch cancer hospital reported that it was common to give muscle relaxants in order to kill those in morphine-induced comas for the relief of pain without their prior consent or that of their families (who were not, in any case, informed about this practice). In short, the evidence suggests that, at best, the present practice in the Netherlands has laid the groundwork for a severely slippery slope. At worst—which I am convinced is already the case—the slide down that slope has begun.[19]

We cannot expect otherwise from efforts to manage the practice of euthanasia. By its very nature, euthanasia would be hard to regulate under any circumstances. It begins with a discussion between doctor and patient in the privacy of the doctor-patient relationship. Their agreement on euthanasia will be known to no one else, unless they choose to reveal it. The possibility of regulating euthanasia depends, at bottom, on the willingness of doctors to report it voluntarily. They are the gatekeepers of the necessary information on the practice. Fear of prosecution, or of professional sanctions, could in principle provide strong inducements for doctors to make such reports, though they have not had that effect in Holland. But if doctors are willing to run some slight risk of prosecution, and if there are no strong oversight mechanisms in place, and if there is an indifference on the part of the authorities to find out exactly what goes on in private, regulations become meaningless. The Dutch situation is a regulatory Potemkin Village, a great façade hiding non-enforcement.

Supporters of euthanasia, using a right of self-determination as their principal argument, can well ask: what right has the state to set itself between a doctor and his patient, much less to tell the patient what conditions must be met for the doctor to perform euthanasia? The Dutch euthanasia situation suggests that such an outcome has already come about. Doctors and patients make their decisions in private and act in private. They do not report to anyone what has been done. Why should we be surprised? Euthanasia cannot in the end be effectively controlled by legal means. Short of putting a policeman in every doctor's office, there is no possible way of knowing what doctors and patients decide to do except insofar as they are willing to make that known. It is a mistake to believe otherwise.

There is a peculiar irony in the contention that, in cases of severe suffering, our human dignity can only be achieved by having another person kill us, or by providing us with the means to kill ourselves. It is a way of saying that we cannot achieve dignity on our own in some circumstances, but must turn to the community to make it possible, at least to one other person to make it physically possible, and the society more generally to make it legally possible. Yet it is a strange kind of community that would require consensual homicide to realize its members' individual dignity. The actual results would be to harm both the individual and the community. It would harm the individual by predicating his dignity and final self-determination on the right to be killed by another. It would harm the community by introducing consenting-adult killing as a means of relieving suffering.

By assuming that the relief of suffering is a goal important enough to legitimate killing as a way of achieving it, we corrupt the idea of such relief as a social goal and duty. We cease helping to bear one another's suffering, but eliminate altogether the person who suffers. We thereby jeopardize both the future of self-determination and the kind of community that furthers its members' capacity to bear one another's suffering. Why bear what can be eliminated altogether? For the sake of controlling the conditions of death, we would introduce a fundamental change in the conditions of living a life. In the name of controlling our mortality, we would enter a claim to change the nature of human relationships.

What Kind of Person Do I Want to Be?

To me the arguments I have just given against euthanasia are persuasive. Yet a pause is necessary. I have had enough experience over the years arguing about euthanasia to understand, I think, one point of great importance. People respond differently to the issue because they have different ideas about, and reflect different traditions of, the self, suffering, and what we owe to one another. I know I will not easily convince those who think that, in the name of personal freedom and self-determination, the introduction of euthanasia is worth running some social dangers. They will usually, if pressed, concede the dangers. They also point out, with some force, that freedom is always dangerous, whether of speech, religion, thought, or choice. They can, moreover, note that much of social policy requires the drawing of lines on slippery slopes; every policy is a slippery slope to somewhere. Even though I find such responses ultimately unconvincing, they are not thoughtless. I reject the apocalyptic notion among some opponents of euthanasia that a kind of nasty death train is rolling down the tracks, destined to wipe out the poor, the burdensome, the demented, and the retarded. This view does justice neither to the seriousness of those who believe euthanasia moral (not all of whom are a Dr. Kevorkian or Derek Humphry, the made-to-order villains for an opposition movement to seize upon), nor to the numerous cultural forces that would remain in place to help control such a trend. I am, it should be clear, not willing to run that kind of risk; others are.

There is, then, about this debate a familiar quality: it pits against one another different ways of looking at the world and the self, and different ways of calculating social gains and losses. In this case, the two broadly contending views have their roots in different parts of the same general tradition. It is never easy to resolve such fundamental struggles.

I would like, however, to put forward another question, one that I will work through in some detail in chapter 4, but which can appropriately be first raised here. What kind of person should I *want* to be in asking questions about my right to life and death? To ask such a question is to help clarify to ourselves a point of some significance. What we want for ourselves, what we *ought* to want for ourselves, cannot fail to reflect some picture, or notion, of ourselves as persons. If it does not do so, then there is surely a profound dissonance at work. For we then want, claim, or demand something that we have not rooted in the kind of person we want to be. It stands apart, isolated, from the rest of our lives, the rest of what we try to be.

Yet now that I have said that, my impression is that most people do not in any conscious way try to relate their claims on others, or on society—including their claim to euthanasia or their denial of it—to some coherent, rounded idea of themselves as persons. I did not do so myself until recently. Only when I became uneasy about the conventional boundaries of the common debate did I start wondering if a different approach to the issues could be imagined: that of asking, not about our rights, but about the kind of people we should want to be. In most of my life, I want and demand a great deal of control. Should I not, therefore, want it in my dying? In most of my life, I expect people to help me to avoid pain and suffering if they can, without great harm or inconvenience, do so. Why, then, not expect a doctor to relieve my suffering directly if he can do so?

But I came to feel—though not at first clearly to think—that perhaps I ought not to want to be that kind of person. I came to notice that, in other parts of my life, my desire for maximum control had not always served me well. It did not create a person I could invariably admire. Nor did my expectation that people would serve my needs, however I defined them, seem always admirable either. Should I not have some concern for the kind of people they ought to be? Which of my needs and demands should they be willing to serve? The answer to that question is not self-evident. And how would the fashioning of my demands, to reflect a certain idea of myself as a person, best interact with the life of another, who would have herself to ask what kind of person she should be to meet my demands? The answer to that complex question does not seem self-evident either.

Devising a Peaceful Death: Snares and Dilemmas

I argued at the beginning of this chapter that the turn to euthanasia represents an understandable, even predictable, response to the various obstacles that scientific medicine and the values it has generated place in the way of a peaceful death. The result of those obstacles is often a violent death by technological attenuation, a life and a death drawn out beyond conscionable limits by medical interventions and moral pressure. Those are formidable obstacles, likely to be only partly relieved by advance directives and other techniques of patient self-determination. Yet a movement to institute euthanasia will simply introduce another form of violence, that of consenting-adult killing, too high a price to pay to overcome the dangers of death by technological attenuation. Euthanasia makes an obsession with control, already a source of medical damage, become still more a source of social damage.

In repudiating euthanasia as an acceptable way to a peaceful death, do I not thereby reject the one certain way to ensure such a death for the individual? Do I not put out of reach a death that is quick, painless, and available while a person is still conscious and competent? Do I not thus undercut my own goal, that of a peaceful death for everyone? I will at once grant that my rejection of euthanasia does close off the possibility of one kind of peaceful death. But it ought to be closed off. The peaceful death of individuals ought not to be bought at the risk, exceedingly high if not likely, of significant societal harm. Nor, more subtly but no less surely, should it be bought at the price of feeding an already excessive preoccupation with control, which generates its own pathologies. As much as we need to pursue a peaceful death, even here there are some means to that moral end that are themselves wrong.

We have, then, a terrible dilemma on our hands: medical progress has made it ever harder simply to allow patients to die, naturally, from their underlying diseases; and euthanasia is a dangerous way to solve that problem. The search for a peaceful death, I conclude, becomes much more difficult than we have recognized. I want, in the remainder of this book, to trace a path out of the thicket—not an easy path, but I hope one that is plausible and attractive. It requires a direct grappling with the meaning of death, of the self, and of medical technology. To that task I now turn.

Chapter 4

LIVING WITH THE MORTAL SELF

Every culture carries within it an image of the ideal self. It is usually flattering and ennobling, a picture of what we are to be and to hope for, not what we still are. It is a self-portrait painted from just the right angle, with the filtered sunshine coming through the window, bathing its subjects in the most becoming mixture of shadow and light.

What has been the ideal self of our enlightened medical culture? It has been a self confident of the fruits of medical advancement and hopeful about the still-greater triumphs that lie in the future. It has counted itself blessed in its ability to transcend fatalism, to rise above the long-outdated, superstitious idea that nature, especially human nature, is forever fixed and unalterable. It has taken comfortable pride in the conquest of infectious disease, the lengthening of average life expectancy, the fact that the lame can be made to walk, the blind to see, the deaf to hear, and the dying to be saved.

The ideal self has been, above all, confident in its ability to manage its medical technology. It knows that not all is perfect, that technology does not always do good, or good inexpensively enough, or for enough people. But it is fully persuaded that, given a proper chance, it can get just the right amount of technology at the right time in the right way and at the right cost, never doubting that, since technology is the self's creation, its vassal child, it can always say no, can always stop, can always turn off the switch.

This ideal self has drawn heavily from the larger treasure chest of modern faith and sensibility. No items in that chest have been so prized as self-control and self-direction, and these are ideas that make us readily receptive to the self of the medical ideal. We have come to think that we as individuals are our own invention, not creatures of the state, or convention, or the past. In the idea of self-determination—fashioned on a foundation of vaulting human rights, and the elimination of slavery to fixed notions of the human good—we have written the final charter of freedom. Our bodies are our own, our lives are our own, our fate is our own. No one, not anyone, has a right to control our bodies, define our lives, or declare our fate a piece of community property.

This image of the ideal self has rested on two convictions. One of them, the first and oldest, going back to the eighteenth century, is that nature can be brought under human control, made to do what we want it to do. The other, emerging later but coming to a fine point in the late twentieth century, is our autonomous right to find our own individual way, to control our living and our dying. In the movement to assess and regulate our technologies, and to place in our individual hands through advance directives the right to say no to them, we assert our dominion over them. They will not get the better of us. In the trend toward euthanasia we see the decisive last steps. We make certain our dominance over nature, giving ourselves the last word if our medical arts fail; and we give ourself the last word in our self-determination, reserving to ourselves the right to have our lives ended when we choose them to end.

Recovering the Mortal Self

I believe that view of the self is mistaken. It cannot be sustained, and it ought not to be. To think that we can bend nature wholly to our will, or bend reality to our technological choices, is nothing less than foolish. In the fact of human mortality, nature retains its own imperial independence. If that ideal of the self is bankrupt (even though it retains many still-valuable piecemeal assets), then we need a new one, better able to cope with mortality in the beguiling presence of medical technology. It must be new, because our historical situation is unprecedented, our scientific and technological possibilities for good and ill are unbounded, and our past efforts are so flawed. Yet it can never be wholly new. We must ransack our past to hold on to what is valuable, take from the present what seems to hold promise, and pull from our vision of the future what appears sound and defensible. We must, in any case, begin with the self. The way we shape our personal pictures of our individual possibilities, explain to ourselves the mystery of pain, suffering, and death, and envision how we want to live in the company of others as we work out the medical and moral implications of our mortality, will set the stage for everything else.

I want to offer the rudiments of a fresh ideal of the self, borrowing heavily from some values often pronounced long dead, but seasoning them with a recognition of the way the new medical developments have given us opportunities we will not, and should not, easily relinquish. If there is ever to be the possibility of fashioning a peaceful death for most and not just some of us, that will require a reconstructed view of the self and its stance toward control, more nuanced, more modest, more realistic than the one our contemporary culture has given us.

I suggest we begin that task by specifying two boundaries, two constraints, to the self and its dreams, the one social, the other personal. The social constraint on the self means that its demand for health and its desire to avoid death do not impose ruinous burdens on others, whether family members or the public. The provision of health care is increasingly a communal task. We are medically and economically interdependent. We need, therefore, a picture of the self that is compatible with that mutual dependence. My desire to live ought not, in its claim upon others, to endanger their own claim, or the claim to important social goods other than health. They in turn are similary constrained.

The personal constraint should be the grounding of the self in an understanding of human nature that grasps and takes seriously a fundamental reality: to be human is to be mortal. What does that mean? To be mortal is to live a life that will be marked by illness, injury, aging, decline, and death. That is an ancient and continuing story, but not the whole story. Another reality poses a counterweight. We can now look to medicine to help us avoid illness, to cure it often when we succumb to it, and to relieve its symptoms when it cannot be cured. We can follow commonsense rules to avoid injury, but expect medicine to help us minimize its effects when an accident happens. We can reasonably hope that the decline of our bodies that will come with age can be lessened, delayed, and compensated for. Though we will and must die, we can hope that we will not die sooner than necessary, that our death will not be premature.

The clash of these two realities—that of mortality, and of the relief of the burden of mortality through medicine—defines our problem. How do we develop a self that knows how to live well with the tension of that clash? How can we have hope in medicine to help us live better lives while we know that our lives must come to an end?

Our first task at present is to recapture our mortality, to give it once again a meaningful relation to our lives. Death must be brought to the surface, given its rightful place, brought back inside of life. The fact of its inevitable triumph—its ultimate necessity—must be built into the very definition of medicine, become once again a part of its own mission, a limit to its art that helps define the nature of that art. Mortality must, in turn, be built into the very definition of the self—a self that human beings once understood with some clarity, but that now lives confusedly in the presence of a medicine that can, and will, make constant advances against the cause of death, manipulating and remanipulating its temporary contingency. Contingency struggles against necessity.

The Fragility of Life

There is some guidance here from the ancient Greeks. The classicist William Arrowsmith offers a potent taste of the way they dealt with the tension between contingency and necessity: "Necessity seems to me the crucial center of Greek tragedy, just as Greek tragedy seems to me unique in the firmness and sharpness with which it follows necessity into human action. . . . Call it destiny, call it fate, call it the gods, it hardly matters. Necessity is, first of all, death; but it is also old age, sleep, the reversal of fortune and the dance of life; it is thereby the fact of suffering as well as pleasure, for if we must dance and sleep, we also suffer, age and die."[1]

Under one common reading, the way of wisdom for the Greeks was the acceptance of necessity, and with it the fragile, contingent nature of our lives. Fragility, chance, mortality, destiny—all constitutive of necessity—define the human condition. Necessity is "that set of unalterable, unmanageable facts which we call the human condition."[2] Martha Nussbaum nicely articulates the way in which acceptance of necessity could be given meaning: "Part of the peculiar beauty of *human* excellence just *is* its vulnerability. The tenderness of the plant is not the dazzling hardness of a gem. . . . The contingencies that make praise problematic are also, in some as yet unclear way, constitutive of that which is there for praising. . . . Contingency, an object of terror and loathing, may turn out to be at the same time wonderful, constitutive of what makes a human life beautiful or thrilling."[3] William Arrowsmith makes a similar kind of point: "Where men are freed from the yoke of necessity, their lives cease to be tragic, and with the loss of suffering comes also the loss of dignity and *sophia* [wisdom]. For it is in the struggle with necessity that heroism is born, and even the hero, if he is to accept his humanity, must accept necessity."[4]

Yet it is troubling for us, over two thousand years later, to accept necessity so readily, especially that most necessary of all events, our own death. This is not so much because we are more arrogant, more full of hubris, than were the ancient Greeks, though that may be true enough. More to the point, the emergence of modern science and the technological transformation of nature have persuaded us that "necessity" itself is malleable. Christopher Lasch has nicely phrased it, in characterizing "the whole modern project" as "the conquest of necessity and the substitution of human choice for the blind workings of nature."[5] Or, as the novelist Mary Gordon has noted of our own culture, "The story of America is the story of the escape from fate. Europeans crossed the ocean in order to be free of it. . . . The freedom and autonomy that America is meant to stand for is the attempt to define the self outside of the bruising authority of fate."[6]

We need not heroically accept infant death from infection. That is not part of biological necessity, though our great-grandparents thought it was. We need not tolerate a heart attack in an eighty-year-old. The attack can be averted and, even if it takes place, angioplasty or a bypass procedure can save the person suffering it from a once-certain death. What, then, are the "unalterable, unmanageable facts" about our illnesses? Surely not that they are inevitable and unavoidable. Not one could be counted theoretically unconquerable. This is the heroic part of medicine, the part more like a gem than a flower.

Yet in our own lives we cannot make a self of that kind of heroism. We will die, and we will die of something not yet conquered, *whatever* it is that is not yet conquered. We cannot live a life, or shape a self, based on the visions of scientific medicine. We are now seeing the price to be paid for trying to do so, the growing fear of death at the hands of that medicine.

Thus we are pressed back to take seriously what we have been led to forget: the necessity of accepting our mortality, but now under altered circumstances, those brought us by medical advances.

Images of Mortality

Is there an alternative image of the possibilities before us? Is there a fresh way of managing the balance between chance and necessity, progress and mortality, acceptance of our fate and the need to struggle against it? There is, but I use the word "image" here deliberately. We are here dealing with a level of consciousness deeper than that which can wholly be influenced by our logic and arguments. The appeal has been to our hopes and our desires as much as to our minds. The power of modern medicine resides in its almost magical possibility of offering us a relief from biological necessity, granting us new powers to manage our fate and our destiny, presenting an image of unlimited hope, genuine knowledge, and great progress. It assumes the possibility of dominating, manipulating, and redefining nature and its potencies. This is a powerful and compelling image to a self all too conscious of its fragility.

Yet the image easily becomes an illusion and a mistake, not because it is wholly without foundation, but because it is partial and half blind. What can be put in its place? Can there be an alternative image as powerful and provocative yet, simultaneously, as soothing and reassuring? No. That is too good to be true, and we do not need, nor should we want, a replacement of the same kind. I want to invoke instead an image of the self that is more flexible, less manipulative, more interdependent with others, more open to risk, a self appropriate to a peaceful death. It is an image less soaring in its pretensions, but more demanding in its implications; less fixed in its self-determination, but more insistent on the strength of the self to choose its stance toward nature rather than feel compelled to dominate it.

To pursue that end, I want to explore five ideas, all of which I believe are true:

(1) Self-respect and integrity need not, and ideally ought not, to be grounded in a capacity to control our lives and mortality.

(2) Pain and suffering can make life a misery, but an obsession to manage and be relieved of them can corrupt us.

(3) The richest self is not one that seeks an optimal stage of life but that is protean enough to cope with every stage, whatever it brings.

(4) Human beings will and must be a burden on one another; the flight from dependency is a flight from humanity.

(5) There is no inherent relationship between a control of one's death and the dignity of that death.

1. Losing Control: The Self Undone. There are two satisfactions in good health steadily sustained. One of them is obvious: our bodies do not stand in the way of our shaping a life. In good health the body is, so to speak, transparent. It is there, our unobtrusive servant, quietly and faithfully doing our bidding. The other satisfaction is even more reassuring. Good health gives us a sense of invincibility, a settled conviction that the chaos of illness, the fragility of a body captured by disease, has been held at a distance. Sickness is someone else's problem, not mine. Other bodies go wrong, not mine. Yet illness as such is not necessarily the greatest threat. Its deepest threat lies in its meaning: it is the undeniable token of our precious hold on life. It reminds us that we are human, not gods, that from dust we came and to dust we will return. The proximate terror of illness is that pain and suffering will ruin us. Its ultimate terror is that it reveals our final fate, which is to lose control of our lives, to see the self that is our deepest possession, the center of our being, as perishable.

The seventeenth-century English poet John Donne has left us a powerfully disturbing way to think about this threat to self-integrity. Time, he suggests, will at first appear benign to us. In gestation, in birth, and in early growth and development, the intentions of nature seem friendly. We are as flowers unfolding, our possibilities limitless and growing always stronger. But we soon discover that time is not so friendly after all. Passing illnesses, those from which we recover, give us a hint of grimmer possibilities. The change that gave us life and hope begins to tell a different story, one of decay, dissolution, and eventual death. Time is no longer on our side, bringing new possibilities. It turns against us and will destroy us.[7] Our "dissolution . . . is conceived in these first *changes, quickened* in the *sicknes* it selfe, and *borne* in *death*, which beares date from these first changes."[8] Donne's perception is timeless: "O how manifold, and perplexed a thing, nay, how wanton and various a thing is *ruine* and *destruction*."[9] Exactly. The modern proliferation of degenerative disease in an aging society has increased the manifold, wanton, and variegated forms of ruin and destruction.

What are we to do with the threat to the self that illness and impending death bring? What are we to make of the innate fragility that menace reveals? In another era, we might have embraced fatalism, or a stoicism not far removed from it: accept that which cannot be controlled. But we have been tutored to a different response. From modern medicine has come the message that hope should not be abandoned. Illness and death are not inevitable, at least not necessarily in this way at this time. From our heritage of freedom and a commitment to self-determination have come a complementary message. Our human greatness, the sure sign of our transcendence over dumb nature, is that the self still remains our own, even in its dissolution. Viktor Frankl called that capacity the "last of the human freedoms—to choose one's attitude in any given set of circumstances, to choose one's own way."[10]

Yet we have, in our modern way, stopped short of asking about the meaning and use of that freedom. We claim the freedom, asserting in its name our right to self-determination, but then often fail to ask how best to understand the freedom once it is ours. There is, in particular, a constant conflation of the right of self-definition with the right to act, though they are by no means the same. Our modern view of the self is typically not, as Frankl underscores, to focus on the possibility of choosing an *attitude* when we are unable physically to act. What has come to count too much is that our choices affect *outcomes* in the world; we are at sea when we cannot do so. It is here that the confluence of modern medicine and the modern temperament expresses itself most tellingly. Both eschew passivity, both reject solving problems of illness and death by adopting an interior stance of acceptance, choosing instead action and domination. Our capacity to act, to *do* something, is cherished—something preferably affecting the outer world of nature rather than the inner world of the self.

The idea of a right to self-determination and self-definition is surely not meant to preclude the shaping of our inner life. Far from it. That is understood to be part of the privilege that the right gives us. But that capacity to shape an attitude inwardly is not taken as the interesting or important or meaningful part. That is instead left in the realm of the wholly subjective and idiosyncratic, not far from mere taste, and certainly not a task for shared common discourse.[11] We do not readily talk about how to shape our interior life in the face of death, because we think its meaning to be private, not easily shared or explored with others. Yet of course death is a universal human experience, and it derives its meaning as much from this universality as from the different circumstances of individual lives and deaths.

We do ourselves a great and double harm by focusing the meaning of self-determination, and the shaping of a self, on our capacity to make external choices, to act. One of the present harms is that we collectively, strenuously, and often obsessively, pursue action to damaging ends, working to change the medical reality at a high cost because of our unwillingness or atrophied ability to see how better to live with our medical limitations. The other harm, looking into the future, is the temptation to block the understanding of our mortality still further by interposing the possibility of euthanasia. That way we can go from the aggressive action of a medical domination of reality to the moral domination of the threatened self by means of euthanasia. If our times had not seen so many of our efforts at control and domination of nature come to a bad or an ambiguous end—think of our environmental crisis, if the medical cases are not sufficient to pique the imagination in this respect—we might remain content with thinking that the key to a right to self-determination is the power to do something, to shape and manipulate the world by action. But it should be clear enough that precisely that stance generates many of our worst problems. We have asserted our right to act, and we see the results all around us, a littering of the medical and environmental landscape with the detritus of our very success.

There is, of course, a quick response to those charges: medicine and technology have given us many blessings, and the price of some harm has been well worth paying. That is not a bad reply— if nothing mattered other than finding the right trade-offs, ways of balancing external harms and benefits. Even so, given the widespread fear of death from the ministrations of advanced medical technology, a fear that we will lose control of our selves, we might well wonder if we have gained the better of that balance. Arthur W. Frank, reflecting on the experience of his own cancer treatment, wrote: "Every day society sends us messages that the body can and ought to be controlled. . . . Control is good manners as well as a moral duty. . . . Physicians justifiably think it is their duty to restore, in the name of society, the control that the sick are believed to have lost."[12] This judgment may be too harsh, but the impetus of medicine, not easily resisted by doctors or patients, is to take charge, to believe as a powerful faith that control can be gained if only enough will, thought, and science are exerted. Yet even if control can be gained for a time, it must sooner or later come to an end. A stance toward control that has no place for that inevitable moment, which can only treat it as a defeat—and probably even culpably so, if we looked more closely—cannot do the company of the sick a service. They will tacitly be instructed that they should not lose control, and that it is in their power, with the help of medicine, not to do so. The fear of losing control, however, cannot readily be banished.

The problem with that fear is that it can only partly be dealt with by trying to hold on to the control. The fear itself is as much the problem as the actual loss of control. It bears no necessary relationship in its intensity to the actual fate that awaits us. We can decide to confront fear, to understand that it is part of our situation, learning as best we can to cope with it. Or we can try endlessly to run from it, trying to avoid it, to pretend it can be banished. Yet the very need to run, the intensity of the drive to escape, betrays the force of the fear. Nothing is harder than to deal immediately and directly with that which terrorizes us, but few responses are more invigorating and strengthening for the self than doing just that. Facing up to terror is something we do entirely with and within ourselves. We do not change ourselves in that act of the will, but confront ourselves, taking our full measure as fearful, insecure people. It is the mastery of self, not of the outside world, that brings the deepest satisfaction, and in the end it is the only mastery that is proof against what the world brings. A significant part of that mastery is knowing when to give up a drive to control our fate.

If we think that it is only our right and capacity to act in the face of mortality that can give us self-respect, we have made a mistake. When we listen to the voices of those who have endured the worst that life can bring, a life of concentration camps and organized murder, we can hear them say something of great importance: what enables people to endure, and to do so with dignity and grace, is not their ability to change their circum-stances, but what they make of them; and what they make of them turns on the kind of people they are.[13] They possess a suppleness, not a rigidity, in the face of a loss of power to manage their lives. They find inner resources to replace those denied them from the outside. They do not accept the evil that brought them their fate; they would be the first to want it changed. But, once it is given, they learn how to let their sense of self-possession redeem what they cannot change.

We all know people whose lives, day in and day out, are dominated by a desire to be in charge of themselves, to have life fully under control. They are restless, even angry, when their lives are interrupted by the unexpected event, by that which unsettles their self-managed existence. They cannot readily abide the notion that they must be forced by circumstances to do something they did not choose, did not contract for. Surprise is their enemy. The worst enemies of all are those unexpected demands that other human beings make upon one's life. In many ways, I am such a person, but I do not like that in myself. I can see in those who live differently, whose lives are not an endless drive for control, a better possibility. They show another way, a no less rich alternative, one tested by human experience.

2. Pain and Suffering. We can push our way deeper into this thicket by considering the possible ways of dealing with pain and suffering. I am constantly surprised by the range of responses they invoke, from self-pity and despair to stoic endurance to a mocking gaiety. In my own experience of seeing people burdened with suffering, there seems to be remarkably little correlation between the objective source or cause of the suffering and the response to it. What one person can endure, another cannot. People put up with, and make sense of, pain and suffering in the most unpredictable, remarkable ways.

Save for the variable feelings of fear and dread, human nature as such seems to force no fixed response to suffering, either in the behavior it induces or in the meaning attributed to it. Everything appears to depend upon a wide range of previous experience and present interpretation. The meaning we will attach to pain and suffering is shaped over the course of our lives. Our history, our culture, our personal structure of understanding will all make a difference to this meaning, but they will be blended in different ways in different people. We are not merely passive victims or bystanders in the process. We can over time fashion ourselves as persons who bear trouble quietly, both working to spare others our private pains as far as possible, and also knowing when to let others give us their help and compassion; or we can allow ourselves to be full of rage and anger, determined that, if we must suffer, so must everyone around us. I do not contend that there can be a total mastery of self and character here, but only that we do have the power to lead ourselves in one general direction or another.[14]

When I stub my toe, the pain can be intense, powerfully dominating. I can think of nothing else—indeed, I cannot even think, but merely experience the pain. The kind of person I am will shape the way I respond to that pain, even to how loud or long I cry out. When the pain is part of an illness or the consequence of a serious injury, it begins to take on yet another meaning: it can begin to say something about my fate as a person, and will also serve to help me find out what kind of person I am already. What illness and the threat of death actually do to me or threaten me with is one thing, but what I make of them is a different matter.

We can distinguish between pain and suffering because of that difference. As discussed earlier, pain is something that happens initially to the body. If it is severe enough, it will bring suffering, the sense of dread, fear, or anxiety that carries the pain into a different dimension. Yet, even here, the suffering can be borne if there is the promise of some ultimate relief. As Eric Cassell has noted, "Suffering occurs when an impending destruction of the person is perceived; it continues until the threat of disintegration has passed or until the integrity of the person can be restored in some other manner."[15] First the loss of control of the body, then that of the self, borne downward by the illness, is the source of the greatest suffering. Yet pain and suffering endured for the sake of another, or even as an expected means to one's own ends, can be tolerated.

Why is there a difference? Is not pain just pain, and suffering just suffering? Not at all. They are, and must be, embedded in a context of meaning and attribution. To suffer for a meaningful purpose, to endure pain with an end in view, is not the same as to put up with them when they seem meaningless. A further distinction is necessary here. There can be meaningless suffering set within a meaningless life. Or we can set meaningless suffering within a meaningful life. The suffering is in that latter case not the final absurd indignity of an otherwise empty, unhappy life, even if a suffering unto death. The suffering can still be great, for the self is faced with its ultimate threat. But that kind of suffering, framed by a life otherwise prized and treasured, full of good memories and still marked by strong bonds of love and affection, can be bearable. It is not that the suffering itself nec- essarily has meaning. It is that the life of which it is a part has meaning, and can be tested and threatened, but not destroyed, by suffering. This distinction, I suspect, explains why some peo- ple manage their suffering so much better than others, even when the cause of the suffering, the underlying illness, may be similar to that of others who fare much worse.

What exactly might explain the different individual reactions to pain and suffering? That is not easy to say. We can rarely tell, as outside observers, whether the actual experienced pain of someone is significantly different from what we ourselves might experience in similar circumstances, or whether the discrepant response lies in the psychological response, the meaning attached to it. As Virginia Woolf once put it in trying to understand the absence of a good way of expressing our pain to others: "English, which can express the thoughts of Hamlet and the tragedy of Lear, has no words for the shiver or the headache. . . . The merest schoolgirl when she falls in love has Shakespeare or Keats to speak her mind for her, but let a sufferer try to describe a pain in his head to a doctor and language at once runs dry."[16]

When we move from the realm of pain to that of suffering, where pain's significance is interpreted by the person experienc- ing it, the complexity is increased. The cause of the pain will provide one level of meaning, whether from a short-term or a permanent malady, and whether itself temporary and reversible or permanent and irreversible. The way that pain is then inter- preted within the life span of the pain, so to speak, adds another level. As Eric J. Cassell has put it, "The personal meaning of the disease and its treatment arises from the past as well as the present. If cancer occurs in a patient with self-confidence from past achievements, it may give rise to optimism and a resurgence of strength. Even if it is fatal, the disease may not produce the destruction of the person but, rather, reaffirm his or her indomitability."[17]

Hardly less important is the social meaning of the illness, the response to the patient's condition by family, friends, and others (and, for some, the absence of such people). Pain that lies within illness is further embedded within a self that suffers from the meaning given it. Both the pain and the suffering, moreover, exist within the larger social world of which the patient is a part. Pain and suffering do not simply happen to people. Their meaning and intensity bespeak a complex reality, as much constructed as given, as much malleable as fixed.

Two important implications follow. One of them is that it is open to us to seek, and perhaps to find, some rationale for our suffering. For many religious believers, the idea of redemptive suffering is powerful. Acceptance of suffering, or understanding suffering as part of a religious interpretation of life, can provide a rationale for the suffering. It remains difficult to bear, but it is not meaningless or pointless if wisely understood. For those of us who cannot turn to a religious understanding, matters can be more troublesome. A life that is moving downhill to death, marked by suffering that comes from grasping the coming destruction of the self, sets the stage for a choice, a choice about the interior stance to be taken toward what is happening. I can decide that I want, and demand, the right of control, interpreting my emerging fate as a challenge to my capacity to make of the world what I will, and to make my body the subject of my domination. I can, alternatively, decide that I will bear the suffering, trying to put into it a commitment to endurance, to find, however hard, some meaning in the condition I have decided to accept.

Yet there is something not quite right about the choice understood in that way. Is it plausible that I could become an entirely new person at this point, and thus have a decisively clean choice? That is unlikely. Such a decision would almost certainly reflect some pre-existing attitudes and values. The way I choose will more likely express what I have believed over my life, the kind of person I have wanted to be, and the kind of person my actual pattern of thought and behavior has made me.

If that is so, we must then ask: what kind of a person do I want to bring to my suffering, and to the illness and fear of dying that provoke it? What kind of person ought I *now* to be shaping and nourishing for that encounter? Those are questions no less important than asking myself how I want to die. For I may, in those prior and more basic questions, have already supplied most of the answers for the latter, but will only discover that when I am dying.

I return to a simple human fact: we will all have to endure pain, and we will all suffer at some point, perhaps many, in our lives. That is certain and fixed, the price of being human. But there is nothing certain and fixed about how we will respond to such pain and suffering. That response is not biologically determined. It can, to a considerable degree, be created, shaped, and directed. We are fated to suffer and die. We are not fated to make one interpretation only of this necessity, or one response, or to have just one possibility of shaping the contours of our suffering.

3. Mourning the Loss of the Optimal Self. Although we typically think of pain and suffering as a major reason why some people desire to live no longer, that is not the only reason. Increasingly I hear people say that they want their lives to end when they are "no longer themselves" or "not the kind of people they want to be." They seem to have in their minds some idealized picture of themselves, one that they want to preserve. Is there an optimal self, some point in my own history where I become all that I might best be? What might we make of the idea, held by some, that death should come when their highest state of life has passed, never to be regained?

To think about that question, consider an old puzzle. If immortality were suddenly granted me, at what age would I choose to live forever? If I chose childhood, I would have the possibility of an eternity of wonder and discovery, but also of powerlessness and anxieties. If I chose early adulthood, I would have lasting physical vigor and attractiveness, but not the insight and experience of accumulated years. If I chose late middle age, I would have lost much of the physical vigor and appearance of my earlier years, but would have gained knowledge, confidence, and ripened good sense; my youthful follies would be behind me, and even the worse ones of middle age.

The frustrating part of this imaginative act is that no time of life seems quite right. Each has its pluses and minuses. What should I conclude? There is no optimal time of life and no ideal self that belongs to it. If we observe other people, does there seem to be some stage of life that is happier than others, more satisfying? Not in my observation. Some people make a mess of their youth, but find themselves in their later years. Others glide through their early years, only to run aground as they age. Some elderly people enjoy their freedom and lack of family or job responsibilities; others feel empty and dispossessed.

Now, this might suggest an obvious point: since people are different, each of us could find his or her own optimal time of life, willingly trading off, say, maturity for physical perfection, or vice versa. But even that way of thinking seems to me misplaced. Those, in my judgment, who manage the course of life most effectively are the ones who both savor the benefits of the different stages of life and accept their accompanying burdens with good cheer. They have an optimal self, but it is not one dependent for its sustenance upon their external circumstances, whether age or physical or mental condition. It is instead a self of their own inner making, fashioned from the ingredients of their enduring values and ideals.

When my children were growing up, it took me a long time to realize that what mattered was the possibilities of their daily life as children, not what they would be when they grew up. It is all too tempting to think of children simply as adults-to-be, as if their childhood and teenage years were nothing but preparation for some final high point. It is no less common, of course, for people to think of old age as a fall from grace, with the central and important part of their lives now in the past. The error is the same in both cases—that there is a central, ideal point in the life cycle.

There is not. Each stage can have its magic and its tragedy, its glories and its miseries. The children who delight are those who behave as children, making the most of their possibilities, not sullenly waiting to grow up, as if that were when real life would begin. "Real life" in one sense has no stages. It is just the way life is, here and now. The impressive elderly are those who act just their age, shrewdly organizing their lives to enhance what they can do and to minimize the frustrations over what is no longer possible. They live life day to day, neither regretting the past nor fretting about the future. The ancient who whines that life is not what it was is often enough the same person who whined as a child that it was not yet what it should be, or the middle-aged person who complained that he was losing his hair and trim figure. I once heard someone's elderly grandfather described as a man of great energy and activity who, as he aged, had to live, because of illness and aging, within a smaller and smaller physical radius. Yet, even as that radius narrowed, first to the yard he could not leave, then to the house he could not leave, then to the room he could not leave, and finally to the bed he could not leave, he adapted to each smaller world, making of it with good cheer whatever was possible. An imaginative flower arranger I once heard[18] said that the secret lies in learning how to work with the material at hand, not longing for flowers not available. He then demonstrated what he meant by fashioning a wonderful arrangement from roadside weeds.

Yet we need to push a step further here. We may well recognize the folly of failing to see that each stage in life is life, that one is not necessarily better than the others. But what about losing precisely those capacities that make us a self, that give us an inner life? What about losing our memory, or seeing our intelligence diminish, or finding that, because of various intellectual and emotional deficits, our capacity to interact with other people is severely diminished? We may well and wisely recognize that, though embodied, we are not just our bodies, that we can have a viable self at any age even if our bodies are imperfect. Can we so readily come to terms with the loss of what seems—inwardly, to ourselves—to be the core of that viable self?

No, we cannot. No one could find that tolerable, much less easy, to bear. But it may be no less a mistake to think that we must have an optimal mind than that we must have an optimal body. There were many times when I was happy as a child even though I had little knowledge and little in the way of memories. My ability to think was not the key to my happiness. Now I have more to remember, a lifetime of memories—and I too often cannot recall them. I turn to my wife to ask her for a name, or to remind me of a dinner party even a week ago. Yet I am a better, more astute observer now than I once was. I used to remember more but notice less, and I did not have the years of experience that have seasoned my judgment (though some of that alleged seasoning, I'm sorry to say, can create a more opinionated, not necessarily wiser, judgment). I can still enjoy reading a novel, even if I quickly forget both its title and its content. "What," I ask someone, "was the name of that book I was reading last week, and while you are at it what did I say it was about?" I have come to admire elderly people whose minds and memory are not what they once were but who, with humor and self-censored frustration, make the best of things. I do not, however, want to minimize the tragedy and anguish possible here. The loss of mental faculties is a severe challenge to the self, and cannot perhaps be fully transcended by anyone. Yet some people, obviously enough, manage better than others. Even here there is no fixed biological determinant of how well or badly we respond. That will, in part, be up to us.

As a male, I can well understand the high suicide rate of elderly males who find life burdensome, its point now lost on them. What will I do when I can write no longer, when—to put a point on it—this book will have been forgotten and no others will be forthcoming? Should I consider that the end of my significant life, as may be my inclination? Yet, when I recognize the great discrepancy between elderly male and female suicide rates, some seven to one, I have to wonder.[19] Is what is going on here among males just a rational consideration of life, a thoughtful appraisal (as is our male conceit, of course), or is it perhaps a matter of man's greater dependence upon status, upon job identity, upon the possibility for acting upon the world and having that world deferentially respond?

I think, by contrast, of a once-distinguished engineer, long old and retired, who now finds satisfaction in talking with the superintendent in our apartment building about the technicalities of repairing its decrepit boiler. He is content to be on the sidelines, but lively still in his interest in a world that was once his. There is a protean self, not the one identified some years ago as a modern self without a center, but a more enduring self that, if so allowed by its possessor, can be coping, flexible, accommodating to reality, and capable of small satisfactions, even though it remains altered.

Why should we believe that life is not worth living if the self is not optimal? It can be made worth living by those whose selves are supple enough to adapt to their own limitations. The self that really counts in the long run is the self that finds its own center, knowing that the center must be composed of what is now possible to the self, what it can create from within, not what once was and what might have been.

4. Dependency and the Relief of Suffering. A core ideal of the modern self is to be independent and self-sufficient, not dependent upon the help of others. "I don't want to be dependent upon my children," my mother would constantly say, echoing a twentieth-century middle-class ideal of self-sufficiency. A no less powerful notion is that we have a duty to relieve suffering, perhaps the strongest moral imperative in a secular society. Yet there is a strain when these two commitments are examined side by side. The first ideal presupposes that we can in fact be independent, that it is within our power to be self-sufficient. The second ideal presupposes just the opposite: that human beings suffer, need the help of others, and will be dependent, at least some of the time. Superficially, these notions can be reconciled: we should strive to be independent but, if that fails, we may need the help of others.

I suspect that there is a deeper tension here, however. The individualistic goal of self-sufficiency carries with it a rejection of what has come to seem the cloying, even suffocating, burden of a family and social life that demands we carry, as our own, another's lives and burdens. A common life based upon voluntary contracts (the consenting-adult model of human relations) and self-determined burdens, has come to seem far more attractive. We have looked to medicine, science, and affluence to provide the wherewithal for this individualistic independence. Since illness and debility are a common source of dependency, they should be eradicated. When they are, freedom will be ours, and not only freedom from our own illness, but also from the unwanted burden of others, themselves afflicted with illness. Such has been the modern vision.

That great day, I note, has not arrived. It will never arrive. People will continue to get sick and to suffer and to need one another, and usually in ways that are demanding, inconvenient, and unwanted. What are we to do with the fact of suffering, which throws us on one another's mercy, and which has not yet been banished and never will be? The first line of defense in advanced societies is to look to social programs of one kind or another. We can use our taxes to help relieve us of personal, intimate responsibility to bear the suffering of others; helpers and services can be bought, respite can be found. Yet that does not always work, or it works only for a time. We are left with the fate of another. Then we discover something at once humbling and appalling. We can be with another in his or her suffering, and we can try to share it, but we cannot relieve it. The individuality of suffering, the way it is hidden away in the psyche of another, means that it is, in the end, not wholly open to our ministrations. How could it be? How people respond to the meaning of suffering may, and often will, have little to do with its objective causes. All we can do is talk, or sometimes only be with people in silence, hoping we can affect that meaning. But, finally, even if the rest of us can perhaps lighten the load a bit, it can only be borne by the person whose suffering it is.

If the suffering is accompanied by feebleness, disability, or dementia, the circle closes all the tighter. We are confronted by a troubled, dependent person whose deepest longings—for bodily wholeness and personal independence—can never again be satisfied, and whom we can do little to make whole again. Thus, the admirable goal of relieving suffering has boundaries. It cannot always be relieved, especially when it is the last, the terminal, illness. No less important, the parallel goal of remaining independent can only be achieved for a time. Sooner or later, for a longer or a shorter period, we will all be dependent upon others. At the least, it is a risk that is ever with us, an inescapable part of life.

Why do we treat this as a human disaster, something that must at all costs be banished from the human condition? Why not, instead, understand that a single-minded desire for independence in our own lives, or a drive to relieve fully the suffering of others whatever the cost, can end in a dreadful distortion of our common life? The greatness of human life, its most majestic stories and epics, has not always centered on dramas of triumphant independence, standing alone and isolated in the midst of the crowd, though surely there are many such stories. It has no less often centered on the way people worked to share their suffering, to create bonds of interdependence. The great triumphs of the concentration camps, or the gulag, are not tales of people learning to be independent of one another, or nobly choosing suicide to avoid suffering. They are instead triumphs of endurance, of inward dignity, of "choosing a stance," as Viktor Frankl

put it, in which the interior life compensates for a lack of independence in the exterior life.

The point is not that suffering is a good to be courted in
ourselves, or ignored in others, or that dependence on others is
a condition to be cherished. Suffering is the most vivid manifestation of a self that must deal with its mortality, its transitory
nature, its fragility. We can relieve another's hunger, or physical
pain. But suffering can only be relieved in part, precisely because
the deepest suffering comes from living with the fact of our
mortality, that ultimate danger of annihilation. No other human
being can lift that hazard from us. To attempt to remove that
sense of threat once and for all, to intimate to another that such
suffering need not be borne, is to cut the very soul out of human
life.

Why? Because fragility is our human condition, however much
it may on occasion be masked or temporarily mastered. Even if
we try to hide this from ourselves, we know it nonetheless. There
is just so far we can go in trying not to notice it. To cover it
over, or to ignore it, is to falsify our life, to engage in the worst
kind of self-deception. Its corrosive effect will eat at every aspect
of our lives. If we do not understand the inescapability of our
mortality, we are in a poor position to understand our own anxieties in confronting illness, our relationship to other people and
their suffering, and the way we think about the course and end
of our own lives.

Something similar can be said of an obsessive drive for independence and self-determination. A view of life that sees independence as the highest and most indispensable good is bound
to be impoverished—by its failure to observe our actual human
interdependence, always present but usually invisible and taken
for granted, and by its willingness to understand that there is no
real loss of self in dependence. Only the error of confusing an
inability to control one's action (as distinguished from one's
interior life) with a loss of self altogether, could lead to that
conclusion.

Does the threat of dependence lie in the burden, even the suffering, that we might impose on another? That is a perfectly reasonable concern, but it is not an ultimate human evil that one person must care for another. Harm is not willingly being done to those forced to provide care. One wishes it could be otherwise. But the potential for harm in trying desperately to avoid such an imposition can be great. It is a way of excluding other people from our lives, a way of pretending we can do without them. It bespeaks an attitude that will and must pervade our relationships with others well before death is on its way.

Why can we not bear a self-understanding that would seem to make us less than our own creations, our own possessions? It can only be because the threat of dependence lies in the insult to a self that has created a myth about itself, a myth of separation and transcendence. But it is a myth. We are not separate and transcendent, even if we can achieve these states now and then in our lives. The inevitability of aging and illness means that our individual transcendence of dependency cannot be, and will not be, permanent. It is a profound error to think we are somehow lessened as persons because dependency will happen to us, as if that condition itself *necessarily* robbed us of some crucial part of the self. It does not. There is a valuable and necessary grace in the capacity to be dependent upon others, to be open to their solicitude, to be willing to lean upon their strength and compassion. To be a self is to live with the perpetual tension of dependence and independence. The former is as much a part of us as the latter. The latter may just feel better, and surely flatters us more. It still remains only half the story of our lives, however.

I am not claiming that the relief of suffering as a moral goal is a low value or priority, or that dependence is a condition to be welcomed. Not at all. I want only to work against the assumption that we cannot *possibly* do well by others unless we can relieve their suffering, that we *must* relieve one another's suffering. Equally, I want to argue that, despite the view that dependency upon others is a special harm to the self, it is no such thing. It need not compromise the integrity of the self, nor need it destroy the life of those who must provide care. Both claims rest upon a thin and shriveled notion of our own strengths and possibilities as persons, and the kind of relationship we should have to one another in our mutual suffering.

5. Managing Death: The Self Annihilated. What are we to make of our own death? How are we to understand its place in our lives? It is not enough, as an answer, to say something general about death, something that applies to all human beings. That can be helpful, locating an individual's death within some framework of meaning and explanation. But it is the singularity of my death, its utterly unique and unrepeatable pointedness, that may be most disturbing. The threat of death is not captured by reducing it to its general parts, those parts made up of separation from others, or of the loss of future possibilities, for instance. Each of those parts has a familiar correlate in our ordinary experience of living a life. It is, rather, the entire and irrevocable loss of the self, which has given us a center from which to interpret and manage the world, and of the body, which has enabled us to act in that world, that is unique to death. Even the death of others, which we can observe, is not instructive; it is *their* death, not ours. Nor are there any other analogies to a loss so severe, so final. There is no way we can envision what it means to be dead.

If our imagination cannot accommodate that circumstance, asking us to envision ourselves on the other side of a divide that is inconceivably alien, it can vividly picture the course leading to death, that of dying. We can draw on our other experiences of loss to see in dying a final intensification, a last gathering up, of everything in life that has been most threatening, now focused in one singular event. There may be, at the least, the threat of pain, but now a pain that is final, unpassing. Thus the one thing that often keeps us going in the face of pain will be lost—the hope that it will be relieved in time.

Yet there is a greater threat. If it is not possible to imagine what it means to have lost the self altogether, which is death, it is possible to bring to mind the experience of a disintegrating self. That is a self that is no longer its own master, no longer sure of its own identity, no longer able to envision a future for itself; and now, for that matter, a self whose own coming end is accentuated, driven home, by the body—whose own pain and disintegration aggressively pull the self down with it. Death makes all too clear that we are embodied selves. If we are lucky, our sense of self, our unique identity, may be the last thing to go as the body falls apart. But we may not be lucky, and we will have to watch the entire edifice of life come down before our eyes.

Is it any wonder that we long for control over our dying? We want, we think, to manage the deterioration of the body, the vanishing into nothingness of the self, in ways that make death our creature, fashioned the way we want it. If we cannot alter the ultimate fact that we die, we can at least control how we die. We can make of our death a token of our life, one bent on self-control and self-definition.

I do not want to deny the power of this idea. It says much about the way I want to die and, in its own way, can bring a dignity to death. But great care is needed. It is an ideal that can readily sour:

- when it is thought that a death that lacks self-management cannot be a death with dignity
- when the desire to control our dying becomes a fearful obsession
- when we demand that medicine distort its own best ends to enable us to retain control
- when it becomes a way of evading a confrontation with death and its meaning for our lives
- when organized efforts to control the circumstances of dying legitimate and augment the societal and medical evasion of death

As Leon R. Kass has reminded us, the roots of the idea of dignity lie in what the individual brings to his or her life. Dignity is not something given to us. We create our own dignity: "It is a term of distinction; dignity is not something which, like a nose or navel, is to be expected or found in every living human being. Dignity is, in principle, aristocratic—that is inescapable, quite apart from the way one might specify the content of excellence or distinction. It follows that dignity, thus understood, cannot be demanded or claimed; for it cannot be provided and it is not owed. One has no more *right* to dignity—and hence to dignity in death—than one has to beauty or courage or wisdom, desirable though these may be."[20]

However much we work to control the circumstances of our dying, its essence is the loss of ultimate control, the final disen-franchisement of the controlling self. Our dignity will stem from the way we come to understand and master that loss, not from the loss itself. We evade the full meaning of death if we think it can be redeemed or transformed by control of the details of the dying, as if the careful writing of instructions about our dying, or the choice of a proxy, would lift the weight of dying from us. What we truly need is the capacity to master our dying, which is not the same as controlling it. Mastery requires that our interior self be in charge of itself, even when death is coming and control over the body has been, as it must be, lost.[21] We already mis-understand death if we think that a careful attention to the medical details of dying will nullify its menace to the self. Only a mastery of the self will do that for us, and only with great difficulty, the fruit of a life getting ready.

I say this because I have been struck on occasion by what seemed at first a curious phenomenon: those most obsessed with getting their advance directives just right seem little inclined to think or talk about how they understand their own death. As with the rest of their lives, they focus on management, an or-ganizational problem, that of making certain they get just the kind of treatment, or nontreatment, they want. Perhaps this is not so curious after all. It can be a wonderfully effective way of not thinking about death while ostensibly confronting it.

Patterning a Life, Preparing a Death

How should I want to live in order that I may die well? That question in turn raises many others. What kind of a private person should I want to be in the face of suffering? Tough, enduring, courageous? Or something else? How should I begin to prepare myself for self-mastery, for pain and death? At the same time, how should I think about the social implications of the self I choose and the death to which I aspire? What kind of public person do I want to be in my living and my dying? How should I think about my relationship with others—my family and friends, and then the larger society of which I am a part?

None of us can know with certainty exactly how he or she will respond to the prospect of death, much less if dying is marked by great pain and suffering. The enormous variability in the way people react to pain, and the great range of interpretations brought to suffering, mean that we can little predict the response of others or guess at our own response. Often enough, we should know, what we have been dreading turns out to be less horrible in reality than in our imagination. Often, indeed, the fear is not all that specific. It is a dread of the unknown, filled with inchoate images of pain and distress, that plagues our imagination. Then we discover that we can cope better than we expected. But not always. Sometimes we are unpleasantly surprised by what happens to us. Things can be worse than we anticipated, and it is the surprise itself, the very lack of anticipation, that generates its own terror: since we did not expect this to happen, still worse may be in store for us, as yet incalculable.

That each of us seems to have a special vulnerability, idiosyncratic phobias, enhances the uncertainty. For some it is the dread of actual pain, for others a sense of helplessness, and for still others a deadly fear of suffocating, of not getting enough air (which happens to be my phobia). That imagined terror can be powerful even if the prospect for recovery is good. Yet when it is combined with the likelihood, or certainty, that it has become one's final fate, then the terror takes on a dimension of ultimateness: This is all there is, and there is no more. Should I want to put up with that, and what should I be prepared to accept?

I can see no way to guarantee or control our reaction to the prospect of suffering and dying when it actually comes to us. If we know in advance, however, that our response is not necessarily fixed by nature or biology, then we can begin to shape the self and the person whom we will bring to that experience. How we die will be an expression of how we have wanted to live, and the meaning we find in our dying is likely to be at one with the meaning we have found in our living. As the great essayist Michel de Montaigne wrote: "Fortune appears sometimes purposely to wait for the last year of our lives in order to show us she can overthrow in one moment what she has taken long years to build. . . . In this last scene between ourselves and death, there is no more pretence. We must use plain words, and display such goodness or purity as we have at the bottom of the pot."[22] "If I can," he adds, "I shall keep my death from saying anything that my life has not already said."[23] The great seventeenth-century theologian Jeremy Taylor made a similar point: "And how if you were to die yourself. Only be ready for it by the preparation of a good life. . . . Else there is nothing that can comfort you. . . . For if you fear death, you shall never the more avoid it, but you make it miserable. . . . No man can be a slave but that he fears pain, or fears to die."[24]

We must, over a lifetime, shape the kind of person we want to be, hoping that what we have made of ourselves by the time we must encounter our death will have made us worthy of its sovereign challenge. Since we know, moreover, that the values of the culture around us will make a difference in our response, we must decide how to respond to, and select from, those values. At the heart of the increasingly popular claim for a right to euthanasia, for instance, is the claim of a right to control our fate totally. That is one possible ideal to pursue. We can recognize the source of that ideal and the claim it generates, arising both from some of our legal and moral traditions and from the power of medicine to help us manage our fate. The question is: to what extent should I, in shaping a self, want to accept and try to live out *that* vision of the good of the self? Quite apart from any rights I might have, is a person who looks to, and demands, a right to perfect control of his or her life likely to be a happier person?

Does it always and invariably serve the good of persons to have control over their fate? This has been the great wager of modern individualism, which has bet not only that the mere possession of choice and control is a powerful value in its own right, but also that individuals so possessed will shape better lives, and now, presumably, better deaths as well. Yet why should we believe that? The Roman Stoics held such a view, one that combined resignation in the face of death with a drive to control the process of dying; that tradition has echoes in our own culture of control. There is, however, an alternative view, with roots as rich and deep: that it is our capacity to learn how to accept what life puts before us, to be open to that which we cannot control, and to embrace the virtues of courage and endurance in the face of evil, that constitutes the greatest value of our lives.

The problem with a life dedicated to control, a life dominated by a fear of helplessness and a loss of power, is that no degree of vigilance can ever be sufficient to assure its success. However much we try, we cannot always control or dominate what happens to us. For just that reason, and to avoid the obsessiveness that a desire for full control imposes upon the self, we may well be better served by a stance of openness and acceptance. I do not say that it "will" serve us better. I only say that it "may" do so, but in support of that "may" we can all think of people whose ability to endure and accept in the face of setbacks, tragedy, and pain is admirable and enviable. It is less certain how many people whose lives are dedicated to control turn out to be equally admirable and enviable. Be that as it may, the notion that a fully self-managed life is better prepared for suffering and death could be quite wrong. On the contrary, a person who has learned how to let life go may have not only a richer and more flexible life, but also one that better prepares him for his decline.

I have clearly tilted my analysis and prescription toward the side of the continuum that favors relinquishment and passivity, openness and flexibility vis-à-vis the unwanted and unexpected. I have been nurtured in that bias by the great religious traditions (even though I do not consider myself a religious believer), and by the example of so many people in our own time who, through character and a capacity to transcend persecution, an absence of choice, and a world stacked against them, made something glorious of their lives and their suffering. They did not choose to suffer, and they did not deserve to suffer, but they took that circumstance and created meaning.

Fashioning a Public Self

We do not live alone, nor are we likely to die alone. How we respond to the prospect of death will reflect the values of the society of which we are a part, and of the family and circle of friends that make up our private lives. At the same time, how we act, the way we live and die, will make a difference in the lives of others. They will see us, and our influence will, if only subliminally, affect the way they think about their lives and death. When I speak, then, of "fashioning a public self," I mean both the way we embody and ingest the values of the society around us, and the way we in turn affect it. The relationship, I suggest, is mutual. It is in that sense that our supposedly private decisions are usually quite public, both in the values that inform the private sphere (taken from the outside) and in the implications and lessons that our private choices have for the lives of others.

Few seem to disagree that, if a person has family or other serious social responsibilities, he or she would be morally derelict in committing suicide or demanding euthanasia. Others have a serious moral claim on him. Our supposedly most "private" decisions almost always have a public dimension and generate expanded obligations. Two different sets of such expanded obligations can be discovered, the familial and the civic.

Even if we have no specific moral obligations to family or friends that our death would leave unmet, we must ask ourselves just what others will make of our death. How might it affect their lives? We know, for example, from many studies and personal experience that a suicide in a family usually has a lasting impact, increasing the likelihood of suicide among other family members, and usually leaving a residue of guilt and regret (no matter if the guilt is in no way rational). This only suggests how naïve it is to think that suicide (and even so-called rational suicide) is a wholly "private" matter. We have of course less experience with euthanasia, but it is reasonable to suppose a similar response: it may well leave others feeling bad, even if the euthanasia seemed justifiable. For there is a deep sense in which suicide and euthanasia are likely to represent, at least in part, a failure of the community, whether that of the intimate community of family and friends, or the larger civic community, to respond to the needs of another. It is the premise of suicide-intervention programs, at least, that active efforts to help those who are contemplating suicide can be enormously effective.

An elderly woman, a neighbor but otherwise a complete stranger, committed suicide next door to me when I was ten years old. The memory of her body on the floor, seen through a crowd of policemen, has stayed with me to this day, as has the memory of my childhood family physician, who also took his own life. I do not know what went on in their minds, whether their acts were expressions of despair, or positive acts of choice against an unwanted fate. I only know that I have never forgotten them. Their private deaths had great ramifications for others, even a child at considerable distance. They remain for me the ultimate image of despair, and that is the ultimate sadness and failure of a self.

How should we live a life that will bring out the best in our neighbors, in our fellow citizens? It may be that a life that courageously faces pain, that waives a demand for perfect release, may do so more than a demand to be killed when the suffering seems too great. The fact that we know how subjective the response to suffering is, how much influenced by the actions of others and the values attached to it by families and society, should at least make us attentive. We may be doing harm, holding up for people an image of response to suffering that is less than ideal— indeed, an image that others may make use of, in their own imaginings, in ways that would be debasing and demoralizing.

Control, Choice, and Character

I have tried to explore here the relationship between the desire for control, widespread in our society, and the kind of ideas, many mistaken, that are believed to support it. Everyone will want some degree of control. We none of us like to imagine ourselves utterly deprived of a right and an ability to make choices about our lives, to make our lives our own. We cannot, in any case, live with modern medicine without making choices. Mere passivity and sheer resignation will not do: we can too easily be used and abused. But we can become our own person in our choices, and that person can be someone who sees the subtle but real traps in an overwhelming urge to achieve full and perfect control. My target has been the mistaken belief that a *necessary* condition of our self-worth is our control of our lives. Since the historical record of the human capacity to endure suffering, and on many occasions to ennoble its otherwise evil reality, shows that to be a patently false belief, why have so many come to hold it? A quick, but not wholly satisfactory, explanation is frequently offered. We have become unwilling, in our affluent and comfortable society, to tolerate the thought of any suffering. We want it banished from the human condition and have naïvely thought that possible.

Another, far more disturbing, possibility may explain the obsession with control. We have come, in modern life, to shape
an ideal of the self and its character that is empty of all content
save that of choice. Choice—and the control over life and death
that is its necessary condition—has come to be understood as
the final meaning of human existence: the capacity to make of
ourselves what we want to be. What are the implications for
individual character nourished by such a view? The most obvious
is that the given in life, the unbidden pain and suffering imposed
by the body, can have no meaningful, legitimate place. It is the
enemy, that which stands in the way of the shaping of a self of
our own choice. It is precisely the brute force, the external and
unavoidable nature, of illness and death that make them so
intolerable. When they cannot be overcome, they seem to be
saying something very decisive about the self that we would shape
as we wish: No, you will not—you will have to live with the
body that nature gave you, now disintegrating, and a self that
cannot will this reality away.

We might dearly like to deny that there is a fixed self embedded
in a fixed body, that either possesses an inherent nature. Illness
and death, however, will not allow that. Nothing could be more
given; and even if we look to euthanasia as a way of shaping
that given to allow us some degree of mastery, it has set the basic
premise and context, that we will sicken and die. If we would
like to reject all other notions of an essence of human life, to
make up our own, that is one we cannot reject.

It is an enormous error to act as if the possession of choice
could obviate the need for the kind of individual character necessary either to make good choices when we have them to make,
or to live well and without despair in the absence of choice. We
can only live well without choice if we have become the kind
of person who can be a person while lacking choice. To make
our sense of well-being and dignity dependent upon a capacity
to control and manipulate our circumstances is already to have
set ourselves up for a fall. We will have become the kind of
person who has lost sight of reality, who has found and wallowed

in the ultimate evasion of hard truth, thinking our death cannot be meaningful unless a self-creation or tolerable unless devoid of suffering and self-diminishment.

It is not simply that an unrestrained dedication to gaining control of our destiny may lead us to do things that are wrong and harmful, though that is surely possible. More to the point, such a dedication will make of us the kind of person we ought not want to be, one who has nothing other than the possibility of choice to call his or her own. We should neither want to become such a person ourselves nor advance the ideal of such a person in our society.

Should I want some control over my life and death? Of course. Should I think that I am somehow less of a person when I cannot have that control? No. Should I have a right to specify conditions for the medical management of my dying? Yes. But if I am thereby led to make of myself someone who cannot endure the thought of not having control over death itself, I will have done myself great harm. I will have created a person who, having lost a mastery of the inner self, has now become pathetically dependent upon changing reality in order to find himself. That is not something we should want to happen to us. Reality tends to go its own way, not ours.

Chapter 5

NATURE, DEATH, AND MEANING: SHAPING OUR END

Two conflicting, even contradictory, understandings of death have long held sway. Death, we have been told, is a part of life, to be embraced with grace and dignity. "How beautifully he accepted death," I have heard said. Death is also reputed, no less frequently, to be the enemy of life, to be resisted and rejected. "She fought to the end," I have also heard said of more than one person I've known, and there are few who cannot recall the almost too familiar words of the poet Dylan Thomas, "Do not go gentle into that good night. . . . Rage, rage against the dying of the light."[1]

Which should it be: accept or fight? Most of us have experienced this dilemma, drawn now one way, now the other. That struggle bespeaks radically different stances toward death, each plausible in its own way, each appealing to coherent, albeit mutually conflicting, ways of construing our fate. Why is it so hard to choose between them, at least for most of us? Why are we so often drawn one way, then another? Which way ought we to be drawn? Which way is most likely to prepare us for a peaceful death?

We can, without much difficulty, understand why these are such hard questions, and why the struggle between our conflicting inclinations is so troubling. The struggle pits two elemental realities against each other, both insistent in their claims, each having an inner logic that does not readily make room for the other. One reality is that of our impersonal biological nature, which we share with all living creatures, and out of which we have been fashioned. It brings us both life and death, and has given us no choice about living with that order of things. The other reality is our innate, but highly personal, drive to live, and to shape biological nature to enable us to do so. That drive is as much a part of our human nature as the biological destiny that will bring our lives to an end. The thwarting of this natural drive, and the destruction wrought by death on our lives as individuals and as members of a community, constitute death's most obvious threat.

The working premise of modern medicine has been that there is an answer to this ancient struggle. Illness and death, it has instructed us, should in principle, even if not always in daily medical practice, be resisted and rejected, fought at every turn and with every imaginable scientific skill. Nature is malleable, scientific medicine says. The diseases that cause death can be cured one by one (thus dismantling death itself), the limits of our biological nature can be overcome, and mortality can be pacified. The culture that swaddles modern medicine has also said something of no less importance: the meaning of death in life, that most ancient of human puzzles, can now be put aside. No such effort to comprehend it is now needed. Death has simply been declared the enemy: do not interpret it, banish it! The meaning of death, once so troubling and elusive, has now become the scientific problem of death, to be attacked and mastered. Where that is not possible, then we can at least be given a choice about our death. The quest for a new civil liberty, called a death with dignity, becomes one more way to master death, not as good as banishing it, but a useful standby until that day comes.

It will never come. We must now instead reinterpret death,

seeing if we can devise a more plausible and sensitive understanding than the one modern medicine has inadvertently given us in its fight against it. Now that we can see some of the baneful results of that fight, they should make clear the necessity of restoring the problem of meaning to its rightful place as an abiding human question. What is the meaning of death in our lives? How are we to understand its place in the human and biological order?

Nature as a Guide

Nature brings life, and nature brings death. As Lewis Thomas once nicely wrote: "It is a natural marvel. All of the life of the earth dies, all of the time, in the same volume as the new life that dazzles us each morning, each spring. . . . In our way, we conform as best we can to the rest of nature. The obituary pages tell us of the news that we are dying away, while the birth announcements in finer print, off at the side of the page, inform us of our replacements. . . ."[2] What are we to make of these primitive facts, as simple and hard as anything in our entire human experience? They make perfectly clear that human life is part of biological and organic life more generally, subject to the same laws of generation and decay. They tell us that, however different we may seem from the dead dog by the side of the road, or the dying raccoon discovered outside our door, our fate will be the same as theirs.

But if nature has at least that much to tell us, does it offer any more helpful insights, of a kind that might be built upon for either understanding, guidance, or even consolation? Most higher mammals, we can observe, seem to die quickly, often from accident or predation by other animals, but also from disease. Their deaths seem relatively peaceful, relatively fast, at least in comparison with the extended death that has become the human lot. Nature in the rough is not notably tolerant of weakness and vulnerability. It seizes upon them to bring life to a rapid end. That was once, we might recollect, also the human way, when death by infectious disease was more common. We might regret that we do not die so easily now, and envy those animals who can die with greater dispatch and ease. Yet we cannot so readily regret the medical advances that turned back those infectious diseases, which rid us of the grossly premature deaths of earlier times.

Do we have it better than the animals? Most of us would say yes, in part because we are not wholly victims of capricious death any longer. Some mastery has been achieved. Nor would we care to be vulnerable once again to those diseases that carried off so many children and young people, making most deaths what we would now think of as premature.

When we look to nature, then, for some guidance, its signposts are not revelatory of much clear meaning. The problem, the obvious problem, is that we are human beings, not just any other organic creature, even if we share with them, our partners in death, many other aspects of organic life. There would be a nice symmetry if nature, which gives us life and takes it from us, also provided us with a way of understanding and accepting that fact, showing us that this is the best of all mortal worlds. But it does not, at least directly.

Yet nature is not wholly opaque. There are some helpful things we can learn from it. The most important is the most easily overlooked: that nature is there, that it brings us all to an end, and that an insensitive effort to dominate and remake nature in attempting to dominate death can easily turn into a disaster.

Our task is the complex one of working back and forth between the biological necessity of death, about which nature does instruct us, and the contingency of death, which is reflected both in the power of medicine to modify, manipulate, and forestall death, and in our human capacity to interpret death in our lives. Both the necessity and the contingency are true, and the question is how to understand those juxtaposed truths, the one constantly wrestling with the other.

I find it helpful here to think of the interpretation of nature much as a sculptor perceives a piece of stone that may be turned into a statue. If the stone is to be shaped into something pleasing and meaningful, the sculptor must constantly work with two considerations in mind. On the one hand, there are an almost unlimited number of ways that the stone can be worked, subject only to the sculptor's inventiveness. That is why the art of sculpture can, like medicine, be forever new, open to fresh ideas. On the other hand, however, the sculptor must know how to work with the qualities and traits of the stone. He must know its breaking point, its relative hardness, its capacity to be polished, its general sensitivity to shaping. If he fails to take those features into account, he risks ruining the stone altogether, shattering it by using inappropriate techniques in trying to shape it, or producing a flawed piece of work, one at odds with its own material.

Human beings are in an analogous situation with death. It can be shaped to human ends and purposes, and medicine has brilliantly done that. But if the nature and boundaries of human and organic life are not carefully considered, and an understanding of them is not part of the creative task, then the results can be harmful or disastrous. The art of managing human mortality will require moving back and forth between possibility and constraint, openness and limits, control and acceptance. That is the understanding of nature I want to pursue here.

The Meaning of Death

What *is* death? How might we best understand death in its own right? The dictionary defines it as "the complete and permanent cessation of all vital functions in a living creature, the end of life." That of course is an accurate, if inert, definition. It lacks precisely what interests us as people destined to die, the meaning of that inevitable biological state of affairs for the person within, the self that is both mind and body, spirit or consciousness and matter, that deep and secret me that neither asked to be born nor, once born, ordinarily asks to die.

The Fear of Death. One way to begin to get at that meaning is to look at one of our most basic experiences: why do we fear death? There is at once something strange here. Nature, which makes it possible for us, in our birth, to exist at all, to live and enjoy a life, takes that life from us; and before doing so, it ordinarily makes us sick and old. Other animals, as far as we can tell, have no problem with this arrangement. We know they react to pain, but we have no reason to believe that they fear death. Why, then, is death a special problem for humans, of all creatures, a problem invoking fear, dread, wonder?

The fear of death is multilayered, not a single response. It gets blended, moreover, with a fear of critical illness and dying, and the borderline is unclear. One of the layers encompasses fear of extreme, obliterating pain and discomfort. Pain can come in many forms—steady, grinding, and predictable, or fluctuating and unpredictable, among others.[3] Its variety is testimony to its tortuous ingenuity. Still another layer is the threat to the self posed by death, the threat of the self's dissolving and the body's coming apart. Pain may bring on this dissolution, or it may come with the dementia or loss of self-awareness of a mind brought low by a body that is ceasing to be. At its heart is the sense that the self is losing its identity, its "I" and a "me" becoming harder and harder to locate.

When the self begins to fade or disintegrate, the loss of a relationship with other people soon follows. Our social world, together with our sense of interior unity and self-awareness, makes us the persons we are. The fear of losing that social world is still another layer in the fear of death. We will lose those whom we love and who love us, never hear their voices again or feel their touch. The dread of deprivation here can be as great as that of the loss of self, and perhaps all the more so if the pleasures and delights of the self entailed living and being with others (as, I think, they should have). We can know as well what our loss will mean to others, to those who love us and live with us, how a part of them will, with our death, cease to exist. We can anticipate their grief and sense of loss, feeling the difference our absence will make to them. A part of their selves will disintegrate in parallel with our own. We can suffer grievously over that, feeling as helpless to help them as we are to help ourselves.

Why must this be our burden? Why *must* our human nature have to put up with these insults? That ancient sense of anguish uncovers still another layer of the fear of dying. We want to know what death means, what kind of a world and what kind of a life make death integral to life. Why should it be *this* way? How can we make sense of things? How can we find ways to justify, or make tolerable, the deprivation that death brings with it, and the dread, pain, and suffering that the course of dying on the way to death provokes?

These are serious, ultimately troubling questions, sometimes called religious, sometimes philosophical. However named, they are forced upon us by the prospect of death. I have no doubt that these questions afflict people with different intensity, and of course provoke different responses. But for every reflective person they are unavoidable. Death can seem a gross injustice, depriving one person but not another of a loved one; or a destructive blow against a self that may have struggled for a lifetime to compose itself and has yet quite to find its way; or the shattering of an inimitably glorious relationship formed over many years in a shared life. How can anyone fail to take such things seriously, or to wonder about the nature of our existence in the face of them?

Is Death a Generic Evil? I have laid out some different, and ordinarily overlapping, layers in our characteristic fears about death. But does our ordinary fear of death, and the fact that dying can be fearsome, mean that death itself is an evil? If so, what kind of an evil? Those might seem strange questions to raise. If death and the dying that precedes it can bring pain, suffering, loss of self, and the deprivation of life with others, what else could they be but evil?

In the early nineteenth century, the essayist William Hazlitt tried to suggest one way of diminishing our fear: "Perhaps the best cure for the fear of death is to reflect that life has a beginning as well as an end. There was a time when we were not: this gives us no concern—why then should it trouble us that a time will come when we shall cease to be?"[4] This is not helpful. Before we were born, there was no one to experience life, no grasp of the goods of life. After a life has been lived, we know what there is to lose, and we know what we will never have again. To be oblivious to a loss does not make it any less of a loss, and the anticipation of the loss of life before that happens is itself a real source of fear. Well it might be, if we prize our life.

We could, alternatively, adopt a stance often associated with the ancient Greeks and Romans: If we cease to exist with death, we will thus experience no sense of loss; our longing for life and meaning will disappear with our death. If there is pain associated with dying, it is temporary and can be borne. Only the loss of virtue and self-respect can really hurt us. A bad dying cannot do harm to a good life.[5] That is too easy a way out. It does not do justice to our recoil from pain and suffering, or to our desire, while still alive, to make sense of our coming death, or to our loss of connection with others. The loss that death brings to our present lives we fear as much as or more than what it might bring us in the future.

Another, characteristically modern, response is more attractive. Death is a necessary condition for the renewal and fecundity of life. It is a source of vitality, change, and complexity. We can hardly conceive of nature without death, at least a nature as rich and generative as the nature we now know. Understood that way, death cannot be said to be generically evil. It serves an indispensable and irreplaceable purpose.

Yet it is not wholly appealing to give a purely biological answer to the question of death. One can say, as I will, that death is a part of the biological life cycle and that, indeed, death is a positive resource for the vigor and continuation of the species. That may well be true enough, but it does not respond to *my* individual self-consciousness and sense of uniqueness, or to my sense of unique vulnerability. My place in the ongoing drama of the species does not capture my enthusiastic allegiance. I did not, after all, choose to be part of that drama. My personal life matters, the life that is mine and mine alone, not impersonally replaceable by future generations of like-gened kinds. No more satisfying is an understanding of death that does not try to plumb its meaning at all, but preaches stoicism in the face of it—the advice given in Bambi, that we must learn to be alone, and to be alone with a meaningless death.[6]

The tension between our status as biological creatures—captives against our will of the generic death-dealing laws of biology common to all organisms—and our idiosyncratic, unrepeatable self-consciousness and will to live, makes death a terrible problem for us. Whether we see this tension as two-dimensional, our singular self counterpoised against our biological universality, or three-dimensional, a push or longing for religious transcendence dividing even that singular self, we are still fragmented creatures, the different parts of our nature in an endless struggle with one another.

Our singular self is one of longings and possibilities, a self that, living in the present, has the potentiality for a future. We are, in that sense, our possibilities, not simply what we happen to be at any given moment. The greatest of those possibilities is threefold: a life of reason, of feeling and emotion, and of relationship with others. Time is our hope as well as our enemy. It provides the continuity for us to fulfill and develop as selves, as well as the entropy that will deprive us finally of our selves. Death may be understood as an evil just because, with it, all possibility ends; there is no future, only a past, and even the memory of that past is to be taken from us.

Yet we cannot interpret death as an evil without a correlative interpretation of life. We may have no trouble agreeing that life is good, or at least (if we are pessimistic) open to the possibility of good. The more pressing question is: what kind of good? Is it an intrinsic good, such that life itself is to be sought and embraced regardless of the harm it may bring to us?[7] Or is it a contingent good—that is, a good dependent upon the circumstances of life? If we take the former view, death will be an intrinsic evil (even if not necessarily the greatest evil humans may suffer), whereas, if we take the latter, then our judgment about death will be a function of the conditions under which it takes place.

There is a middle way open here. Life itself can be judged a great and intrinsic good, the greatest natural good there is. It provides the possibility of creativity and generativity, of realizing an almost unimaginable range of knowledge, feeling, relationships, wonder, and desire. Death is, for the individual, the end of those possibilities. That is not easy to rationalize, so decisive is the loss, so irrevocable what is lost. Yet our experience instructs us that, for those same individuals, there can be conditions of life—illness and decline, pain and suffering the most obvious— that can make life oppressive and destructive, seeming to mock the possibilities for good that it embodies. For some, this will happen because of a specific illness or bodily disaster. For others, usually the very old, it may come out of a sense that life has lost its savor, that its course has been run, that death is appropriate. Neither condition should be thought of as despair, though that is surely possible. More to the point is that the good of life has now been robbed of precisely that which leads us to call it good in the first place, the possibilities it affords us. When they are gone, there can be little left of life worth prizing.

Yet, in the end, we cannot fully understand our death even if we can persuade ourselves to accept it. The experience of life, of its possibilities and its harms, is of supreme value. To them we can only counterpoise nonexistence and ask, as a variant on an old joke, what has nonexistence ever done for me? The paradox, of course, is that we must be alive to curse the burden of life, and if we are dead we cannot enjoy the fruits of life. Only if we understand life to be a good and death to be an evil can it make sense to us to speak of some deaths as more tolerable than others.

If we must die, then better that it should be after we have achieved most of life's possibilities than before. But it would be even better, all things being equal, if those possibilities could continue. It is hard to see how we can prize the joys and satisfactions of life without, simultaneously, wanting them to go on.

Meaning: Perfect and Imperfect

Can we find meaning in this situation, in this human and biological arrangement that so thoroughly mixes together the good and the evil? In using the term "meaning," I want to encompass three elements: our way of understanding and explaining our human situation; the value we attach to our lives; and the sense of emotional wholeness and integrity we experience, the way in which the cognitive and the valuative blend together.[8] All three ingredients are necessary. If we cannot understand by means of some kind of explanation why life is the way it is, we are bound to feel victims of a pointless and cruel world. If we do not have some way of valuing our lives and the world in which they are set, we will not know what to cherish or desire; our lives will have no goals, a terrible situation. Unless we can blend our thinking and feeling and wanting into some integrated whole, we will find ourselves torn apart—our reason fighting our values—with nothing adding up in our interior lives.

Our sense of meaning, however, need not be perfect or complete. We might speak of finding a "perfect meaning" of life: a fully satisfying, coherent way of thinking and feeling about life and death, so much so that we could say, and mean, that this is the best of all possible worlds. That is a high, and I believe unachievable, goal. We might, however, discover "imperfect meaning," by which I mean a likely, more or less coherent view that does justice to much though not all of our experience. I will put forward such a view here, underscoring that it will not be fully satisfying; it cannot be—but it may be the best we can do.

My way into this imperfect meaning will be to return to the

struggle noted at the beginning of the chapter, the tension be-tween our inclination to fight death and to accept death. Death, I contend, can be given a meaning, though imperfectly, if we find a way to understand it as a "part of life." That phrase is by now little more than a slogan, yet, unless we can give it some depth and substance, rescuing it from its pious conventionality, there can be no meaning in death. For there is at work in this struggle about fighting or accepting death a deep and basic kind of dualism: death understood to have a place within life, so that life itself cannot be fully grasped without an appreciation of the role of death; or death understood as outside of life, alien and hostile to it, a meaningless intruder.

Despite the casual talk in our culture of death as a "part of life," I believe that, in reality, the dominant view is actually that of death as an outsider. Modern medicine tacitly embodies this view. As the late theologian Arthur C. McGill acutely noted, death in the medical view is "the instant life ends. . . . Death is something future. . . . As long as we are, then there is no death. . . . *Death in this narrow sense is known primarily by other people.* Death is a future event of our visible nature, out ahead of us somewhere."[9]

Thus viewed, death is fragmented, part of an understanding of life that sees it as divided into two distinct phases, one of which is life itself and the other death; and death is outside of life, wholly separate from life. Because of this fragmentation, death is simply and clearly the enemy to be vanquished or, as a better image, the enemy that must be kept outside the walls, not allowed into the province of life. This general stance has been mirrored in other streams of modern thought. The philosopher Jean-Paul Sartre portrayed death as separate from, and alien to, our lives.[10] It is not that toward which life tends, as Martin Heidegger thought, but is instead a total discontinuity with all that has preceded it. It just cuts off all of life, revealing in the process nothing whatever about the meaning of that life. For Thomas Nagel, death thwarts an "essentially open-ended possible future." Death is thus "an elaborate cancellation of indefinitely extensive possible goods."[11] In this view, there is no way to make death acceptable.

Modern medicine stands close to Sartre and Nagel in its understanding of death, but then adds its own grace note to that interpretation: the possibility of using science and technology to keep that alien and foreign death at bay. We should, with Dylan Thomas, "rage against the dying of the light," but now do so not merely with feeling and rhetoric but with the power of science to change those biological conditions that bring death into life. The pursuit of indefinitely extended life—a necessary good if death is a necessary evil—becomes the logical aim of medical science, which, for its part, has no reason to believe such a good is not attainable.

The alternative possibility is to see whether some meaning can be given to the idea of death as a more integral feature of life itself, not just its outer, external boundary. Unlike birth, which initiates the life of a child within the human community, and can clearly be spoken of as a part of life, death is the end of possibility. Before you die, you are still a human being among human beings. Death puts you decisively and irrevocably outside the human community. The moment after you have died, there is nothing left but a decaying body and a memory in the minds of others. How can that which ends life, death, and which describes a state of affairs that exists when life is no more, be understood as a part of life?

There is a way of interpreting life that can give an integral place to death. I will call it the "continuous," or "inside," view, to distinguish it from the "fragmented," or "outside," view. It begins with a different kind of question. We should not ask whether death is an evil (for this already fragments death), but whether a life course that includes death at its end is an evil. And the answer to this question, in the continuous view, is: not necessarily. It can be interpreted in a more benign way, even if not wholly so.

I quoted Arthur C. McGill above on the medical, fragmented

view of death. The continuous view (my term, not his) he expressed as follows: "Death is not some future event observable
primarily by someone else. Death is going on within us all the
time. Every time we are sick we hear from within what death
shall mean to us personally. Illness is a foretaste of death; it is
the concrete experience where each of us discovers how our own
experience becomes impossible. Every separation from a loved
one is a foretaste of death. Every evening, every letting go of
the conscious world in sleep is a foretaste of death. . . . From
this perspective, death is not some objective event about which
we can be forewarned by our physicians. *Death is the losing of life,
that wearing away which goes on all the time.*"[12] McGill quotes a
pointed comment of Michael Frankel in the same vein: "We
never know death. We know only the little deaths we die as our
years fall away from us, leaving their work of sundering and
separation. . . ."[13] Jeremy Taylor, in the seventeenth century,
reflected a similar view when he wrote: "So is the age of every
day a beginning of death, and the night composing us to sleep
bids us go to our lesser rest; because that night, which is the end
of the preceding day is but a lesser death. . . . And when the
last day of dying will come, we know not. There is nothing then
added but the circumstance of sicknesse, which also happens
many times before."[14]

The Continuity of Life and Death

I will define the continuous view of death as one that contains
two important elements. One of them is an understanding of
death as an event that is ever foreshadowed during life, a life
made up of many "little deaths." The other is an understanding
that life and death are inextricably intertwined, and that much
of the value of life comes because of this relationship, not despite
it. In this view, life itself requires, for its meaning and piquancy,
death as its necessary complement. Life cannot be life as we
understand it without death's being integral to it. Life, moreover,

can only have a trajectory and possibility of meaningful completion if we incorporate the necessity of death within it.
"Death," Hans Jonas has written, "is coextensive with life. . . .
Mortality [is] an essential attribute of life as such. . . . Two
meanings merge in the term *mortal*: that the creature *can* die, is
exposed to the constant possibility of death; and that, eventually,
it *must* die, is destined for the ultimate necessity of death. In
the continual possibility I place the burden, in the ultimate
necessity the blessing of mortality."[15]

The plausibility of this account lies in its capacity to catch a
central feature of our experienced life, that of the constant tension and interdependence of the goods and ills of life, the pleasures and pains. "Feeling," Jonas notes, "lies open to pain as well
as pleasure, its keenness cutting both ways; lust has its match in
anguish, desire in fear; purpose is either attained or thwarted,
and the capacity for enjoying the one is the same as that of
suffering for the other."[16] For human life generally, the same
poignant combination of opposites appears: "Just as mortality
finds its compensation in natality, conversely natality gets its
scope from mortality: the dying of the old makes place for the
young."[17]

There is an obvious objection to be raised here. Even if we
can see a way in which life and death are joined, a way in which
death is thus a part of life, why should we judge this arrangement
to be acceptable? Why should we bless this way of organizing a
universe and the human life within it? Is that the best cosmic
and organic combination that can be imagined? One reason for
accepting it, perhaps unpleasantly realistic, is this: that is the
way things are, and you had better accept it.

A more subtle, more tolerable reason has been advanced by
Irving Singer in his splendid book *Meaning in Life: The Creation
of Value*. We may not, he notes, be able to find out what "the"
meaning of life is, and there may not even be "the" meaning.
But it is open to us to construct *a* coherent and plausible meaning,
to make of the interdependency of life and death something of
value. It is, he argues, part of our nature to be able to find and

create meaning and value, to make sense of what otherwise might seem impenetrable. We can open up creative possibilities, adding structure to chaos. This trait becomes all the more valuable when the world as it is refuses to convey any obvious sense of meaning. "Most people," Singer writes, "realize that death is one of the major facts of their life. And when we live our lives with a genuine recognition of this particular fact . . . giving life meaning *because* we know that we will die in the not-too-distant future, death ceases to be a meaningless termination. It will not have solved or resolved anything, but it exists as a constraint that reveals what it is to be alive as human beings are."[18]

Singer effectively reminds us of two related perspectives, the one manifest in a familiar passage from Shakespeare, the other revealed in a less known reflection of the American philosopher George Santayana. In Shakespeare's *Cymbeline*, there is the song of Guiderius:

> *Fear no more the heat o' the sun,*
>   *Nor the furious winter's rages;*
> *Thou thy worldy task hast done,*
>   *Home art gone, and ta'en thy wages:*
> *Golden lads and girls all must,*
>   *As chimney-sweepers, come to dust.*

In Singer's interpretation of this passage, death is understood as a "relevant completion" of life, and to support this he notes a later phrase from the same play, that of death as a "quiet consummation" of life. Speaking for himself, Singer says: "I am not proposing that death always, or often, occurs as a happy ending. I am not saying that in itself it gives life meaning. I only want to leave open the possibility that we can live in such a way that death has an appropriate, and therefore meaningful, place in our being."[19]

I join Singer's reflection to that proposed by Hans Jonas, and find in a passage of Santayana also quoted by Singer the possibility of added bite and coherence to what I have called the "continuous" view of the interrelationship of life and death: "That the end of life should be death may be sad: yet what other end can anything have? The end of an evening party is to go to bed; but its use is to gather congenial people together, that they may pass the time pleasantly. An invitation to the dance is not rendered ironical because the dance cannot last forever. . . . The transitoriness of things is essential to their physical being, and not at all sad in itself. . . . Folly on the contrary imagines that any scent is worth following, that we have an infinite nature, or no nature in particular, that life begins without obligations and can do business without capital, and that the will is vacuously free, instead of being a specific burden and a tight hereditary knot to be unravelled."[20]

The ideology of modern medicine has come implicitly to hold that we humans have an "infinite nature." It believes that science will help us uncover life's biological secrets and, in the process, help us create endless ways to keep death outside of life. Yet the alternative view, that life and death are continuous, not fragmented, offers a better foundation, both for understanding our lives and for fashioning appropriate goals for medical science. It recognizes both that meaning can be created and it is of our nature to do just that, and that the idea of individual life as finite is biologically understandable and can be made humanly meaningful, if not always satisfying, as well.

Even if we can come this far, however, some serious problems remain. Although we might be inclined to do so, it is not altogether possible to push aside the matter of "the" meaning of life. We might well enough understand how some kind of coherent sense can be derived from a biological world that makes death an integral part of life. Yet we might still feel the terrible pull of our individual lives and consciousness, revolting against a too-passive acceptance of this arrangement. Why this world, and not another? Is this the best imaginable world? Not quite.

The late theologian Paul Ramsey spoke eloquently against the view that death should be seen as a part of life. He argued against what he saw as a too-casual, insufficiently serious invocation of "death with dignity," and against rhapsodic notions of death as a "beautiful event." He noted that death should be understood as the *end* of time for a person, not simply a phase in the passage of time. "Death," he wrote, "means the conquest of the time of our lives—even though we never experience the nothingness which is natural death. 'Awareness of death' means awareness of *that*; and awareness of that constitutes an experience of ultimate indignity in and to the awareness of the self who is dying. . . . Talk about death as a fact or a reality seasonally recurring in life with birth or planting, maturity and growth, may after all not be very rational. It smacks more of whistling before the darkness descends, and an attempt to brainwash one's contemporaries to accept a very feeble philosophy of life and death."[21]

I can offer no easy way out of the choice I have tried to portray here: either accept the notion that sense can be made of death as part of a biological life that must come to an end (the view of Singer, Jonas, and Santayana), or see it as the ultimate insult, not admitting of a satisfactory meaning, to be struggled against and not accepted (the view of modern medicine and of Paul Ramsey). The latter view will not accept the possibility that "a" meaning can be found in death; only "the" meaning is worth pursuing, by way of either conquest (science) or religion (Ramsey).

"There is," Ramsey wrote, "grief over death which no human agency can alleviate."[22] He is right about that, and the inability of nature, for all its rhythms and necessities, to restore to us the person who has died speaks directly to the evil of death for human beings. Death irrevocably assaults the human community. In the cause of biological diversity and renewal, it directly attacks the consciousness of individuality and mutuality that binds human beings who live together as social creatures. I must leave the matter at that. For myself, I am able to live with—for I can do no better—the view that death is a part of life, to be accepted, and the grief that goes with it, to be endured.

Death as Biological and Moral Evil

Here I want to focus on some serious problems that arise even
if we are inclined to accept the possibility of finding some general
and generic meaning in the present biological arrangement. If
we accept the notion that there is *some* meaning to be discovered,
making death in general acceptable, does that necessarily mean
that each and every human death is equally acceptable? Can we,
with some plausibility, say that, even within this world where
death has an essential place and part, some individual deaths are
wrong and evil, and that those deaths should be resisted?

We can and should. I want to speak here of the existence of
such deaths as a "biological evil," on the one hand, and as a
"moral evil," on the other. In these two senses of evil, we can
see the great difference between the kind of tame death celebrated by Philippe Ariès, which seems to admit of no modifi-
cation, and the peaceful death that I want to espouse, which
does. Medicine allows us to fight some deaths, and with medicine
have come some moral standards about when death should be
fought.

Death can rightly be called a biological evil when its timing
and circumstances are wrong. By the "timing" of death I mean
the place of death in the life cycle, which moves through time
from birth to death. It represents, put visually, the horizontal
plane of death. It is in the context of that horizontal plane that
we speak, most commonly, of a person's death as premature or
untimely. Such a death comes before it need have or should
have. By the "circumstances" of death I mean those conditions
that determine the impact of death upon a person and our evaluation of them. Among the conditions, most notably, will be the
extent to which, where possible, a patient has been given some
choice about his death, the extent to which the process of dying
has been accompanied by pain and suffering, and the relationship
of the dying person to the community of which he is a part.
These circumstances will represent the vertical plane of death.

Death is ordinarily a biological evil when it comes well prior to a full life cycle—that is, when its timing is wrong. A full life cycle is usually needed to realize the widest possibilities of individual flourishing and participation in the life of society. The possibility of working out our own lives and their meaning, of developing deep human relationships and life with others, of seeing our own talents bloom and make a contribution to a social life in common, takes time, many years. Obviously enough, as the lives of many great people show, it is not necessary to live into old age to make a telling human contribution; some people achieve that rapidly. Nor is it necessary to live an indefinitely long life to do so. There is no evidence that a longer life *as such* proportionately increases the chances of individual fulfillment or societal benefit. Yet apart from those two extremes, a premature death significantly lessens one's chances of doing what is possible. The death of a child is accounted a great evil both because of the devastating blow to the parents, who lose its love and presence, and because of the loss of possibility for the child, the further development that would have filled out and shaped its life.

Death is also a biological evil when its circumstances are wrong. An accident is the most evident kind of wrong circumstance, for it is, by definition, something that need not have happened and that, with due care, should not have happened. It is a misfortune for human life that comes from the outside; its fault and cause do not lie within the body. An accident may, as with a teenage highway death, be a premature death as well. But even an accidental death in old age may be counted an evil if it need not have happened and interrupts a life still in full flower. An accidental death that comes when death from disease is threatening, a death that might have been much worse, can still be considered evil, especially if it deprives a person of time to put his or her life in order and to allow a proper leavetaking from others.

The circumstances of death are wrong when the dying person is forced to endure extended pain and suffering or is forced out of participation in the human community by a failure of the mind well before the death of the body (as in severe dementia or persistent vegetative state [PVS]). What I want to capture here is the situation where death not only ends life, which can be bad enough in many cases, but where the dying itself destroys the person long in advance of the event of death. It is the deforming of the process of dying, which I will examine at greater length in the next chapter, that characterizes its evil circumstances.

In describing various forms of death as biological evils, I am assuming the truth of an ancient viewpoint, that we can discern some natural goods and ends. Though often challenged by modern philosophy, we still do speak meaningfully and tellingly of "premature" deaths, and of deaths that thwart the full flourishing of human possibility. We do so because we can discern a general trajectory of human life, see what it means to live out a full cycle, and because our emotions, by no means wholly irrational, seem to confirm that discernment. The death of a young person, for instance, will trigger a kind of grief not characteristic of the loss of life of an older person. It is not that the value of the life of the older person is less than that of the younger person, but that we respond to the difference in the achievement of life's possibilities.

Death as a Moral Evil

Death is a moral evil when the timing and circumstances of deaths subject to human influence are culpably wrong. By "culpably wrong" I mean that the deaths ought not to have occurred and need not have occurred, and that some human being was responsible for their occurrence. The simple omission of a human action that might have preserved life cannot, in any sense, be thought of as a biological cause of the death. People usually die of natural causes, not omitted human actions. It is the body that fails them, not other human beings. What matters is our moral judgment about the timing and circumstances of such deaths, that part within human control.

Yet it is a peculiar kind of moral judgment we are asked to make: we seem to have more power and obligation than we actually do. Because death is biologically inevitable and necessary given our organic nature, there can be nothing whatever wrong about allowing someone, at *some* point, to die. It will happen and must happen in any case, whatever we do. Our power is thus radically limited, a fact systematically overlooked in our bemusement over the limited power we do have.

Our moral problem is to determine when that point has been reached. I earlier suggested (chapter 1) that the idea of some decisive moment at which it may be said that someone is dying, or that a disease is terminal, is becoming less and less useful as a standard for making decisions to terminate treatment. The notion that there is such a moment was reassuring. A plausible biological standard was thereby postulated. But with the improvements in medical technology, it becomes harder and harder to make use of such a norm; and medicine is, moreover, able to keep a body from being captured by death long after the person has, through dementia or coma, left the human community as a conscious participant.

We are left with an increasingly tenuous relationship between the biology of death and the morality of intervention into death, but not an absent one. We can determine when the process of dying is deformed, something other than it might be. The dying of a person can be said to be morally wrong when human choice, with knowledge of likely consequences, is responsible for attenuating dying with no benefit to the patient. Dying can also be said to be morally wrong when it is against the wishes of the dying person and could be prevented; when it is the result of deliberate violence, as in murder or negligent manslaughter, or medical negligence; and when it could have been prevented without overriding harm to the dying person.

We can also, simultaneously, go at the matter by looking at the timing and circumstances of death in the life of a person. A death will in general be morally wrong in its timing if it is deliberately allowed to take place prematurely, that is, with wrong timing in the life cycle; and in general morally wrong in its circumstances when these are inappropriate, such as when there still exists a solid potential for meaningful rationality, self-awareness and feeling, and relationships with others. When we are determining our moral obligations to respect life and to struggle against death, our moral judgment should focus on the *timing* and *circumstances* of death, which we can to some extent manage and control, not on the existence of death, which we cannot. If we begin this way, we will at once put aside some confusions and mistakes I have tried to describe, particularly the mistaken view of nature that would have us "killing" those whom we with moral legitimacy would cease treating.

To focus moral judgment on the timing and circumstances of death also helps make clear the way in which that judgment is superimposed by us upon the underlying natural reality of death. We cannot change or alter the finality or inevitability of death, only some of its conditions. We can be responsible only for those conditions, and the moral rules pertinent to them are for us to determine and invent—in accordance with what we think are appropriate goals of human life and pertinent correlative ends of medicine.

In this way, we can break the stranglehold of the idea of medical progress and the technological imperative on the principle of the sanctity of life. The sanctity of life does not require endless medical progress or the use of unrelenting technology to keep people alive. Nor can the value of technological progress automatically call upon the principle of the sanctity of life to provide it with endless legitimation. Whatever it is that we should value in life, it should not be made a function of what medical science renders possible. Whatever it is that we should value in technology cannot wholly be dominated by its efficacy in preserving life.

I spoke earlier of the transformation of death from a biological event only (in the days of prescientific medicine) to a moral event, which came about when there was the possibility of shaping and influencing the course of dying. It was then that medicine, as part of our culture, began creating a moral superstructure for death, developing rules and codes pertinent to that influence. We also began to go awry at that point, not in the development of such rules, but when we began to think that our rules encompassed the managing of death itself, not just its timing and circumstances.

Perhaps we ought not to accept death as part of the human condition and, rather, continue to judge it evil. But it does not follow that we should endlessly pursue medical remedies against diseases that cause death. Since there will always be *some* cause of death, this would be a losing struggle, and necessarily so. That might not matter—"Is not the good fight worth fighting?" some might reply—but for the result it engenders: an unrelenting scientific struggle against death comes to take the place of an effort to understand death, and to develop a medicine that knows how to coexist with it.

Yet where are we to locate the burden of proof when there is doubt about the quality of life and the prospects for efficacious treatment? The yoking of sanctity of life and the technological imperative has led to the common conclusion that, when in doubt, we should treat. Yet since continuing medical progress increases the occasions of doubt—for a treatment with low probability of success in general may work with this particular patient—it will become harder and harder to know when to stop, and thus more and more likely that all death will be considered a human responsibility, not a natural event.

Neither of these two problems of the "quality of life"—that of our supposed obligation always to improve it, or of where the burden of proof is to lie in the presence of doubt—can be adequately addressed without some independent standards about the acceptability of death. Here I want only to establish the kind of timing and circumstances that might allow us to judge a death morally wrong. But even this preliminary foray cannot be fully meaningful without raising, from still a different vantage point, the question of when, if death is not to be judged an evil in its timing and circumstances, it might be termed acceptable.

When Is Death Acceptable?

Is it possible to say, at one and the same time, that death is a generic evil for individual human life, but that not all individual deaths are evil? One way of saying this is to see death in some situations as a lesser evil than continued life. If the continued life is no more than a respirating body, or a life that has lost all potential for human flourishing, we may judge death as a lesser evil than continued life. But is a "lesser evil" standard strong enough? I think not. Some will think that any life under any condition is better than no life at all, and such a position only feeds slavery to a technology that can always keep a body going just a bit longer.

Death is acceptable, I contend, when it comes at the point in a life when (1) further efforts to defer dying are likely to deform the process of dying, or when (2) there is a good fit between the biological inevitability of death in general and the particular timing and circumstances of that death in the life of an individual. This dual standard does not imply that there is a perfect moment for death to occur; that may be an unnecessary fiction. It is necessary to think only in terms of death's falling within an acceptable *range* of possibilities.

Here our ordinary language, well rooted in the past experience of death, is still a decent guide. A death is "premature" in its timing when a person dies either in youth or well before old age, *notably* earlier than biologically necessary. A death is "merciful" in its circumstances, or a "blessing," when in the life being lived the possibility of enjoying the goods of life has been forever lost. A death is "tragic" not only because its circumstances are terrible, but also because it may leave a terrible mark on other people: the accidental death of a child or a young parent, for instance.

All definitions have boundary problems, and so do mine. What does "significantly earlier than biologically necessary" mean, particularly when we do not really know what the biological limits of an individual human life might be? The life cycle can be understood to encompass a range of possibilities, not a fixed portion. Only when we fall short of this range altogether can we feel rightly cheated in our dying. Whereas a person who dies now at the age of sixty-three (my age) might be said to be unlucky in dying in early old age rather than later old age, or prior to the average life expectancy of seventy-five, it would be strange to think of a death at age sixty-three as comparable in its tragedy and unacceptability to the death of a child. The reason for the difference is evident: Sixty-three years is a full, although not necessarily a totally full, life cycle. It is sufficient time to accomplish most of what can be accomplished in a typical life, although more might be accomplished by a particular individual.

I mean by "accomplished" here not the achievement of projects and tasks, but the experience of the goods of living a life. It is not a standard of productivity, but a standard of lived and experienced life. My point, in any case, is that we are not biologically wronged if we die at that age, even though we might be luckier if we can live longer. If there is a wrong, it is that we have been given such a biological nature at all, one that must die. But, within *that* context, a somewhat earlier rather than a somewhat later death is not a biological evil.

Yet a time line based on the life cycle will not itself quite suffice, even if it helps us locate a biological framework for making judgments about the place of death in the life cycle and allows us to speak of a premature death. Individual possibilities count as well. An individual death ought to be considered acceptable when it does not thwart the possibility of further significant development and self-manifestation. That possibility may be thwarted either by a terminal illness, or by an illness (e.g., advanced dementia) that has destroyed or almost destroyed the integrity of the self or personhood. Care is needed here in working with this specification. Of its nature, death means the end of the self and thus of any future self-manifestation; that is why it is, while biologically inevitable, an evil for human life. But within the context of that unavoidable fate, the deaths that typically concern us are those that occur well prior to the end of the life cycle.

Yet are all premature deaths—that is, deaths early in the life cycle—wrong? Not necessarily. They are not wrong when the biological condition of the body will, as the price of its continuance, impose great pain or severe, intolerable disability (though they *would* be wrong if they were against the will of the persons in that state). They are not wrong when a continuation of life will deform the process of dying. The body has, in that respect, lost its own future. We may consider it, properly, a great wrong that someone has suffered such a fate—but not a great wrong, *under those circumstances*, that death will relieve the person of further suffering. It is an even greater wrong to distort the end of life, and diminish the possibility of a peaceful death, by trying to extend life under such conditions.

Yet, even so, suffering may be endured, and further life chosen. Many people elect to live that way, and we often admire them for their endurance and courage. The real end of human possibility comes when the self has no future, when the self loses its potentiality for being a self. What does that require? To be a self, one must have the possibility of self-consciousness (ordinarily encompassing thinking and feeling) and the capacity to interact with others. The death of the self occurs when that potentiality is lost, when the self has no future. The point of having a healthy body is to maintain a viable self, one with the capacity for self-awareness, and with the possibility of self-manifestation and interaction with others. Death should not be considered unacceptable—if death there must be at all—when significant possibilities have been lost.

There is that word "significant" again. Can it be defined? Not with any precision, in great part because there can be serious and legitimate disagreement, which may be unresolvable, about how much of a self one needs to be considered alive in any meaningful sense of the term. Great precision, as Aristotle long ago reminded us, is not to be expected in matters that do not admit of it, and this is surely such a case. Thus, again, I will have recourse to a range: death ought to be considered acceptable if most, though not necessarily all, capacity for selfhood has been lost. It is preferable, in fact, for death to occur *before*, not after, all self-capacity has been lost. Only under those circumstances can a person properly prepare for death and take stock of its meaning, a circumstance requiring self-awareness.

Two other tests, both requiring imagination, can be suggested. One of them can be called the "historical mourning test." Imagine a specific condition—say, that of severe dementia—where a person has not spoken to another person for a considerable period of time or given any evidence of an inner life. Our nursing homes are filled with many such people. If such a person had died of a routine urinary-tract infection a century ago, it is unlikely that death would have been raged against as unfair, wrong, or untimely. Such a death would, we know, have been accepted as the ordinary way in which a person in that state died, and understood as a blessing, a relief, and a release.

Should the fact that we now have inexpensive and effective antibiotics available to treat such infections change that earlier historical judgment about the value of continuing life? Could its omission not be seen as a convenient way of getting an elderly person to die? I suppose someone could bring to such a situation an attitude of expediency, looking to the benefits of the caretaker rather than the sick person; everything good can be corrupted. But if the intention is to do what is right for the patient—the ordinary medical stance—then there is no automatic reason to presume such expediency. If we judge that the death by routine infection a century ago for a person with advanced dementia was not untimely, no tragedy, there is no reason to think it less timely, or more tragic, now, just because we have an antibiotic that might avert it. I contend that the person living in that earlier time was more fortunate, when there was no possible temptation to extend that life. Death in such a situation falls within the range of a good coincidence of the biological inevitability of death in general and the timeliness of death for an individual. More time is not likely to offer a better life, but it will almost certainly increase the likelihood of a poor death.

My other suggested test, a complementary one, I will call the "treatment-invention test." Imagine ourselves back a century ago. An individual is in a persistent vegetative state (PVS), of the kind suffered by Karen Ann Quinlan and Nancy Cruzan, unable to take food or water by mouth. One hundred years ago, that incapacity would, with a permanently unconscious person, have been considered a symptom or manifestation that the person was dying. Would we have wished for the invention of artificial feeding for the *sole purpose* of keeping that person alive? Would we have pined for a technology that could suspend someone in an irreversible PVS state for five, or ten, or even thirty-seven years, as has happened in one case? The artificial methods of feeding now available, moreover, were developed as temporary bridges for people recovering from some forms of illness and surgery, not to keep alive bodies without selves as permanently preserved zombies.

Not all peaceful deaths, of course, are necessarily acceptable deaths. By an "acceptable" death I mean one that is neither biologically nor morally wrong. A death that comes at the wrong time or in the wrong circumstances, even if it is peaceful, is not acceptable. Death ought to be acceptable when (1) it is no longer untimely or premature—and we have no obligation to redefine those terms continually in the light of scientific possibility; and (2) when the circumstances of death are commensurate with the respect we ought to pay to human life—and such value should not be dependent upon the technological possibility of manipulating those circumstances. My goal here is to find a way of taking seriously in medical research and practice—which means also in the culture at large—the biological inevitability of death, which remains unaltered by scientific progress. If we start with that inevitability as our point of departure, not with the malleability of the timing and circumstances of death, we will be better positioned to deal well with them.

I return to my sculptor analogy. The first task of the sculptor, if he is working with stone, is to understand that his medium is stone, not wood or clay or something else. In treating the human body, medicine must for its part understand from the outset that the human body dies, and thus that medicine must, in its sculpting aspirations, be built around this fact, as much as around the fact of malleability and plasticity in the timing and circumstances of death. Just as the sculptor can, so to speak, harm the stone by ignoring its innate characteristics, so too can medicine do harm by ignoring some biological constraints.

The achievement of a peaceful death should not be a goal sought only when nothing more can be done to preserve life or maintain a decent quality of life, when all else fails. It should, instead, be central to the mission of medicine, present from the outset of life and not just at its end. It is a moral evil to distort death negligently by human intervention, just as it is a moral evil willfully to allow death to occur when the timing and circumstances are wrong. The violence inflicted upon a person by murder makes for an unacceptable death. A death that might have been preventable, that takes place at the wrong time and under the wrong circumstances, is unacceptable. A death that comes against the will of the dying person, whether from the commission of violence or the omission of appropriate medicine, is unacceptable.

Yet a death is acceptable if, like a well-wrought statue, it has been fashioned within the constraints and limits of the material with which medicine must work. In this case, the most obvious constraint is that of the biological inevitability of death. A death should be morally acceptable if medicine has taken that inevitability as one of its starting points and has sought a death that does not transform our dying into something it need not be. Death is also morally acceptable if, in thinking about timing and circumstances, medicine has sought to enhance life but not at the cost of deforming death. It is acceptable if it has not extended life past its potential for human personhood. It is acceptable if it has not come at the cost of technological brinkmanship, which threatens a decent life as much as it promises to preserve it. It is, above all, acceptable if it recognizes that the value, or sanctity, of life does not depend upon what medicine can do to improve or extend it. Human life is sacred because it is the source of human consciousness, which can be enhanced and often protected by medicine, but is not dependent upon medicine as its final protector.

Chapter 6

PURSUING A PEACEFUL
DEATH

On the face of it, one might be forgiven for thinking that death
at the hands of modern technological medicine should be a far
more benign, sensitive event than death in earlier times. Do we
not have a much greater biological knowledge, thus enabling
more precise prognoses of death? Do we not have more powerful
analgesics, thereby enhancing the capacity to control pain? Do
we not possess more sophisticated machines, capable of better
managing organs gone awry? Do we not have greater psychological knowledge, suitable to relieve the anxieties and suffering of
an anticipated death? Do we not, adding all that up, have at
hand exactly what we need to enhance the possibility of a peaceful death?

The answer in each case is yes and no. Yes, we do have much
more knowledge than we did prior to modern medicine. But no,
that knowledge has not made death a more peaceful event, either
in reality or in anticipation. The enhanced biological knowledge
and technological skill have served to make our dying all the
more problematic: harder to predict, more difficult to manage,
the source of more moral dilemmas and nasty choices, and spir-

itually (if I may use the term) more productive of anguish, ambivalence, and uncertainty. In part this is because, with the
advent of modern medicine, the earlier superstructure of meaning
and ritual was dismantled, thus setting death adrift in a world
of uncertain values and import. But, also in part, it is because
modern medicine brought with it a stance toward death that is
ambivalent about its necessity and inevitability.

The technologies of medicine, ever more clever in their ability
to sustain failing organs, provide a set of tools that endlessly
sustain this ambivalence and allow it to be played out in tortuous
detail. Precisely because they have opened up new possibilities
in the ancient struggle with our mortality, those technologies
have made our understanding of mortality all the more difficult.
To confound us further, they have misled us into thinking we
have a greater dominance over our mortality than earlier people
had.

What can be done to gain a better way of thinking about
medical technology and our human mortality? How can that
technology be made to serve a peaceful death, not to be its
enemy? What can be done to bring about a change? I want to
try to make plausible a different way of thinking about the use
of technology, and then suggest some ways of implementing it.
The change I propose can be put very simply, however strange
and odd it may sound: death should be seen as the necessary and
inevitable end point of medical care.

Death as the End Point of Medical Care

In considering its appropriate goals, medicine should, so to speak,
simultaneously work backward as well as forward. Medicine now
characteristically works forward only, looking to promote the
good of life, both to lengthen life and to improve its quality.
Death is reluctantly admitted into the clinical realm of medicine
as the limit to achieving those ends, but that limit is itself uncertain at its boundary, not readily located. Thus also is the

termination of treatment judged to be a lesser moral evil, because the quality of life cannot be sustained at the level at which, ideally, medicine would like to sustain it.

What if, however, we began our thinking with death? What if we asked how medicine should conduct itself to promote both a good life and a peaceful death? What if medicine finally accepted death as a limit that cannot be overcome and used that limit as an indispensable focal point in thinking about illness and disease? The reality of death as a part of our biological life would be seen, not as a discordant note in the search for health and well-being, but as the foreseeable end point of its enterprise, and its pacification as a proper goal of medicine from the outset. What if the aim of scientific medicine was not an endless struggle against death, with the fight against disease as the token of that struggle, but helping humans best live a mortal, not an immortal, life?

These questions are almost naïve. But I see no evidence that they are deeply and persistently asked in modern medicine. If they were, death would have to be taken seriously, its limiting and circumscribing place allowed full entrance into the ideals of medicine, not treated as only a necessary evil and an instance of scientific failure. The acceptance, management, and understanding of death would become as fully a part of the mainline enterprise of medicine as the pursuit of health. It would not be necessary even to conceive of a hospice movement, a separate system of caring for the dying; that would be taken for granted as central to the enterprise of medicine itself, not a specially constructed side show, out of sight of the main tent.

If the ordinary goal of medicine is the preservation or restoration of health, death should be the understood and expected ultimate outcome of that effort, implicitly and inherently there from the start. The only question is when and how, not whether. Medicine's pursuit of health should be leavened by its need—when health fails, as it must—to prepare the way for as peaceful a death as possible. If death is part of the human life cycle, care for the dying body must be integral to the ends of medicine.

Death is, to sharpen the point, that to which medical care should be oriented from the outset in the case of all serious, potentially life-threatening illnesses, or of a serious decline of mental and physical capacities as a result of age or disease. Of each serious illness—especially with the elderly—a question should be asked and a possibility entertained: could it be that this illness is the one that either will be fatal, or—since some disease must be fatal—should soon be *allowed* to be fatal? If so, a different strategy toward it should come immediately into play, an effort to seek a peaceful death rather than fight for a cure.

What am I saying that is different from the present stance of medicine? That stance now takes as its sole task the pursuit of health, or the preservation of a decent quality of life, with death as the accidental result of illnesses and diseases thought to be avoidable and contingent, even though in fact still fatal. Death is what happens when medicine fails, and is thus outside its proper scientific scope. That is why, I surmise, a great medical classic, *Cecil Textbook of Medicine,* a primary guide for physicians, refers directly in fewer than twenty-five of its twenty-three hundred pages to death (and only in five to pain).[1] This book, filled with accounts of lethal diseases and ways to treat them, is strikingly silent on treating patients in the terminal phase of those diseases, giving three pages only to the topic. And those pages are isolated from the diseases that bring death. The slighting is a stark example of the way death is kept beyond the borders of medicine, an unwelcome, unwanted, unexpected, and ultimately accidental intruder. What if, by contrast, every section of the book dealing with potentially fatal diseases had a part dealing with the care of people dying from the disease? Even though there are many similarities, the care of the dying cancer patient is not identical with that of a person dying from congestive heart disease or kidney failure. But this could never be guessed from reading standard treatment textbooks.

An incorporation of that approach in textbooks and clinical training would make clear, in the most direct way, that *this* disease may be, sometimes voluntarily and sometimes not, the cause of death—death, which must come to all and is thus no accident. Then the physician's task would become that of accepting a particular illness as the likely cause of death, opening the way for a peaceful death by choosing the combination of treatment and palliation of the accepted condition most likely to make it possible. The objective here would be exactly the opposite of technological brinkmanship, which goes as far as possible with aggressive treatment, stopping only when it is useless to go further. In the former case, brinkmanship would be repudiated from the outset. Active treatment to cure disease and prevent death would stop well *short* of its technical possibilities, at the point where a peaceful death could be most assured and best managed. The worry that a patient might die *sooner* than technologically necessary would be effectively balanced by anxiety that a patient might die *later* than was compatible with a peaceful death.

To make what I am saying clear and plausible, two general steps are necessary. I shall first specify some minimally necessary conditions for a peaceful death, and then sketch the kind of moral and medical context necessary to enhance its possibility. Four pieces must now be put in place as part of the initial step. First, I will specify more fully the nature and components of a peaceful death, noting along the way how our dying can become deformed. Second, it is necessary to reintegrate illness and death, now torn asunder by technological interventions. Third, a way must be found to alter a basic moral presumption of contemporary medicine: when in doubt, treat. Fourth, the different possible stages for stopping treatment need to be specified, with a consideration of the appropriate medical treatment for each of those stages.

Deforming Our Dying

A peaceful death can be understood both positively and negatively. I will begin with the latter, specifying some ways in which our dying can be deformed. If we can better discern some of the ways that happens, the ideal of a peaceful death can be given greater substance. Our dying can be deformed in three ways: by deforming the process of dying, by deforming the dying self, and by deforming the community of the living.

Deforming the Process of Dying.   The process of dying is deformed when it is subject to the violence of technological attenuation, unduly extended by medical interventions, directly or indirectly.

Technological brinkmanship is the most common way of creating the deformity—that is, pushing aggressive treatment as far as it can go in the hope that it can be stopped at just the right moment if it turns out to be futile. That brinkmanship, and the gamble it represents, can both save life and ruin dying; this is the dilemma it poses. The most obvious kind of technological violence comes when a particular course of treatment—some forms of chemotherapy for cancer, say, or cardiopulmonary resuscitation (CPR) for a dying person—itself directly imposes the violence.

Less noticed, but bound to become increasingly important, is the inadvertent violence done when the cure of one disease sets the stage for the advent of another, perhaps even more cruel than the former cause of death. Consider, for instance, the person cured of cancer at seventy-five who is set up for the enhanced risk, by virtue of age alone, of the onset of a fatal case of Alzheimer's disease at eighty, or for an excessively long period of severe frailty. We increase the likelihood of spending our declining years helpless, demented, and incontinent if medicine helps save our lives long enough to help us avert all of the lethal diseases that stand in the way of that (not so splendid) final outcome.

We may, of course, gain some extra good years before that happens, and for some it will not happen at all. I only want to underscore the gamble implicit here, a kind of technological Russian roulette with one's last years of life. We must reckon whether it is a good or a bad gamble, and how much we are prepared to accept a deformed dying as a result. Increasing frailty and bodily decline are themselves part of the aging process, the wasting away that ordinarily precedes death in old age. There is no inherent evil in the dependency that withering can bring. My complaint is instead directed against a kind of medicine that drives us toward technological brinkmanship and thus needlessly exacerbates and attenuates the withering in destructive ways, genuinely deforming the process of dying. The process of dying is deformed when, through overconfidence in our power to man-age technology, and to manage our own ambivalence toward death, we fail to take account of what an overzealous medicine can do to our aging and dying.

The process of dying is also deformed when there is an ex-tended period of a loss of consciousness well before we are actually dead. It is deformed when there is an exceedingly and unduly long period of debility and frailty before death. It is deformed when there is a lengthy period of pain and suffering prior to death. Note the words I have used: "extended," "exceedingly," "unduly," and "lengthy." By this I mean to say both that death may well and unavoidably be preceded by some pain and suffer-ing, some loss of consciousness, some debility and frailty, but that we human beings have generated our own miseries when we allow technology to create a situation that produces exceed-ingly long periods of those evils. I offer no precise definition of "exceedingly." Frailty and debility can be tolerated for longer periods of time than straight pain and suffering, and even a few days of unconsciousness might be tolerable.

It is when those evils go on and on that a problem, a desperate one, arises. Left unattended, the biological process of dying would not *ordinarily* lead to such deformities, even though it would happen in a minority of cases. That is something we can know from the dying of other biological organisms, especially higher animals, and from the historical record of human death itself before our modern era, when an extended period of dying was the exception rather than the rule. Our contemporary deformities of dying, it is then fair to say, ordinarily arise *only* as the result of human medical intervention.

Deforming the Dying Self. The most obvious way in which the dying self can be deformed is by allowing the fear of death, or the fear of what dying may do to our ideal self, itself to corrupt the self. Obsessions with a loss of control, or with a diminishment of the idealized optimal self, or with the prospect of pain, are other ways this can happen. That turns our dying into an occasion of unrelenting self-pity and self-castigation: I can never be again what I once was—I do not want to be what I now am—and I do not want to be what I will become as my death draws even closer.

Some delicacy is in order in trying to make this point. It is understandable that we not want to lose all control, or to become less of a self than we once were, or that we fear pain. Anxiety, even terror, is to be expected as we approach our death, because of the physical threats of dying and also because of its challenge to our sense of self-worth and self-coherence. It is the preoccupation with those evils that introduces the potential deformity, the feeling that we cannot be worthy human beings if they are our fate, and the inability to think of anything but our losses, our failures, our diminution.

Deforming the Community of the Living. Just as we can harm our selves, our sense of self-worth, in responding to the threat of death, so too can we do harm to others. If the horror of death—or, more likely, of illness, decline, and dying together—yields social policies designed to relieve that suffering at all costs, then the community of the living is put at risk. A society that takes the relief of the ordinary burdens of life, of which death is surely one, as a goal to be pursued with singular dedication must ultimately fail, and in so doing must put its members in harm's way.

This can happen when the pursuit of health and the avoidance of death become an excessively high priority, pursued at the cost of ignoring other social evils. It can happen when the medical community comes to believe it must, as the price of relieving suffering, be prepared to kill or assist in suicide, thus distorting its oldest and most central traditions. It can happen when, as a community ideal, a life that includes any suffering is rejected as intolerable. It can happen when a life thought "not worth living" (the Nazi expression) is one marked by suffering, a less than ideal self, and a failure to make adequate social contributions to society.

The possibility of a peaceful death will, then, require as a minimal condition that death not be deformed, either individually or socially. But more will be required to enhance its possibility.

Defining a Peaceful Death

It is not difficult, just listening to the way people talk about the kind of death they would like, to gain a decent sense of what they would count as a peaceful death. I could try to do that, but I would prefer to put it in my own voice, recognizing that there may be individual variations:

• I want to find meaning in my death or, if not a full meaning, a way of reconciling myself to it. Some kind of sense must be made of my mortality.

• I hope to be treated with respect and sympathy, and to find in my dying a physical and spiritual dignity.

• I would like my death to matter to others, to be seen in some larger sense as an evil, a rupturing of human community, even if they understand that my particular death may be preferable to an excessive and prolonged suffering, and even if they understand death to be part of the biological nature of the human species.

• If I do not necessarily want to die in the public way that marked the era of a tame death, with strangers coming in off the streets, I do not want to be abandoned, psychologically ejected from the community, because of my impending death. I want people to be with me, at hand if not in the same room.

• I do not want to be an *undue* burden on others in my dying, though I accept the possibility that I may be some burden. I do not want the end of my life to be the financial or emotional ruination of another life.

• I want to live in a society that does not dread death—at least an ordinary death from disease at a relatively advanced age—and that provides support in its rituals and public practices for comforting the dying and, after death, their friends and families.

• I want to be conscious very near the time of my death, and with my mental and emotional capacities intact. I would be pleased to die in my sleep, but I do not want a prolonged coma prior to my death.

• I hope that my death will be quick, not drawn out.

• I recoil at the prospect of a death marked by pain and suffering, though I hope I will bear it well if that is unavoidable.

There is a difference between this desired peaceful death and Philippe Ariès's tame death. Technological advances make it possible to manage better those conditions that could not, in the past, be made amenable to a tame death, especially the degenerative diseases of aging. We can, that is, have both the advantages of the older tame death and, with the help of technology, many improvements in contemporary death.

The most evident characteristic of a peaceful death as I have outlined it is the way it blends personal, medical, and social strands. Whatever meaning we find in our dying and death must come from within ourselves, though we may and probably will, of course, draw upon religious and other traditions for important help. We could also reasonably look to the larger society for public practices, rituals, and attitudes that can provide a more comforting context for the acceptance of death. A modified return to special symbols of mourning, such as black armbands for men and dark clothes for women, as well as the enhancement of groups organized for grieving spouses, or religious services, would be examples of the possibilities here. As for the relief of pain, there we can look to medical practice, and even expect from that practice some help with suffering, a more subtle condition stemming in part, as discussed earlier, from an interior perception of the significance of dying and from the kind of external support we are given in the face of our anxieties.

Could a peaceful death be assured every patient? No. Medicine cannot now, and probably never will be able to, avert all pain and suffering, or ensure a tranquil course of illness. No society could wholly overcome the fear of death, or the rending of community that death constitutes. No person can be confident that fear, anguish, or a sense of pointlessness and futility will not be his lot, even if he has lived the kind of life most conducive to reducing that possibility. Since no one else can give us, as if it were our own, a meaning to our dying and death, we must find that for ourselves; some of us will never find it.

Because there can be no guarantee that a peaceful death will be ours, some store of courage must be available. If I am correct in my surmise that the obsessively feared loss of control of our dying is itself part of the problem—a fear that we will not be either ourselves or in command of ourselves—then one way to resist the force of this fear is to be willing to accept some loss of control. The price of obsession is undue fear. Relief can be sought in a willingness to live with, and die with, less than perfection here. Yet, if we can understand that there is a middle way, the possibility of a peaceful death can be greatly enhanced. It is at least as likely that we could create the possibility of a peaceful death for a majority of people by changing our medical attitudes and expectations as by the more violent course of euthanasia and assisted suicide, and with far less loss of other values in the process.

Illness and Death

The enormous ambivalence about, and evasion of, death is of course nowhere more evident than in the subtle, tacit distinction that runs through scientific medicine, that illness, and the diseases that cause it, can be distinguished from aging, mortality, and death.

Death can only be brought back within medicine by a repudiation of the mythical line between illness and death. This point must be made with some care. There is surely a logical difference between them. It is clearly possible, moreover, to cure disease, and it is conceivable (if not imminently probable) that many of the most serious present degenerative diseases in aging, from cancer through Alzheimer's, can someday be cured. What cannot be overcome is a twofold barrier: (1) the cure of one lethal disease will require that another take its place as a cause of mortality—as in a zero-sum game, the causes of death can only be moved around, from one condition to another; and (2) each of us will die of a particular illness or incapacity (or some combination of them), not of mortality or aging in general. This is precisely what our aging and mortality set us up to do, creating an unbroken continuum between illness and death. To say this is not to deny that the shifting of the causes of death cannot have benefits, such as increased life expectancy or an improvement in the quality of life. Reducing or retarding illness in the aging is of obvious value. I only want to underscore the obvious: death is never vanquished, and death always comes from some illness.

What we can extract from this hard truth is of great importance for medicine, if it can only take heed: illness must be accepted with the same sense of inevitability as death itself and understood to be at one with death, especially as a person ages. This means that, with each serious illness, the question should be raised whether *this* illness should be allowed to proceed and become the cause of death. The present way of managing the critically ill is ordinarily just the opposite, treating each potentially fatal illness as if it were reversible, and as if it must be reversed.

Instead of thinking, as I propose, that *this* death *now* may be better than another death later, the modern way is always to prefer the later, different, death over the present possibility. This is another variant on the idea of brinkmanship: a deferred evil is always a better choice than a presently accepted evil. But that, of course, is not necessarily true. There is no reason whatever to believe that a later death from an as-yet unknown cause will be better than a death from a present known cause. Perhaps so, perhaps not. I am suggesting instead that, once a potentially fatal illness appears, it be considered seriously as the candidate for the cause of death, if other conditions of the timing and circum-stances of death are acceptable. To be sure, if the illness is one that promises an unpleasant death, more so than from other causes, any sensible person would try to avoid it. But if that is not the case, and the death from this disease might be at least no worse than from other diseases, it should be a candidate as the accepted cause of death.

How are those who choose to die from a lethal disease that has not yet reached its fatal phase to be helped in bearing that choice? How might a physician best explain to a patient the bene-fits and burdens of dying from a particular disease, so as to allow a competent patient to make a reasonable choice? If a patient chooses not to die soon after being diagnosed and with little therapeutic intervention, how might the physician best offer a series of structured, incremental options, allowing the patient to go so far but then stop when futility appeared increasingly likely? Can we, that is, overcome a presumption always to treat?

Changing the Presumption to Treat

There is a deeply embedded presumption in medicine: when life is at stake, there should always be a bias in favor of treatment. This presumption lies at the heart of technological brinkman-ship—which would take treatment as far as it can effectively go; and at the heart of conflation of the technological imperative and the sanctity of life—which together make it seem wrong ever to stop treatment while something further can medically be done. This understandable bias has been well stated by Richard Momeyer: "Assuming everyone's death to be an evil until it is persuasively demonstrated to be at most a lesser evil affords a significantly greater degree of protection to the vulnerable. . . . The analog in the law is that innocence is presumed until guilt is proven."[2] Moreover, apart from protecting the vulnerable, there are strong religious traditions that affirm the moral duty to preserve life, though few that would do so under all circumstances.

Yet although one may accept the power of such considerations, a question must be asked. Does the obligation to preserve life require running the risk that patients will die a wild death? Does it require that we forgo the chance of dying a peaceful death, even if that death would come earlier, *perhaps much earlier*, than one from technological brinkmanship? If, prior to modern medicine, a tame death was biologically possible, even if not universal, must we now risk an unpleasant death in deference to technological possibility or out of respect for life?

I answer no to each of those questions. There can be no obligation to pursue life-extending therapy at the risk of a bad death. On the contrary, the pursuit of a peaceful death is a perfectly legitimate personal goal and a reasonable demand upon medical care. Death is a moral evil when it is willfully chosen as a way of escaping our familial or social obligations, or when it comes violently, without our consent, at the hands of others. It is an evil for the individual as well as society when it comes through euthanasia or assisted suicide, which would create a wrong peaceful death. But death can be seen as morally acceptable when timing and circumstances allow us to avoid unnecessary pain and suffering, to be conscious and alert, and to remain within the circle of human companionship. I call such a death a "moral good" because it allows us to achieve important personal as well as social ends. We are more at one with ourselves and those around us. By contrast, the wild death of technological attenuation, or the personality-destructive death accompanying advanced dementia, alienates us both from ourselves and from those around us.

What about the charge, sometimes leveled, that the present situation, permitting only that patients be "allowed" to die, is itself no less open to abuse than is euthanasia, and perhaps even more so, because harder to detect? Abuse is of course perfectly possible, and indeed difficult to detect when treatment is stopped and death allowed to come. But it is a mistake to see a symmetry between the two situations. Doctors *must* at some point stop treatment. That cannot be escaped. Sooner or later, they can do no more for patients. Ordinarily, they can allow patients to die earlier than possible only if death is already on the way— that is, only in the borderline cases. Euthanasia is, by contrast, never required medically. It is an entirely different kind of action, not only because it directly causes death in a way that stopping treatment does not, but also because it changes radically the institution of medicine and adds a new social occasion for direct killing. Allowing to die is already, of necessity, part of the in-stitution of medicine. Even if there is abuse there, it would be of a different character from that with euthanasia—bad enough, but not as bad.

When should the customary presumption to treat be changed? It could legitimately be changed:

- when there is a likely, not necessarily certain, downward course of an illness, making death a strong probability; failure of more than one organ is an obvious example in an older patient
- when the available treatments for a potentially fatal con-dition entail a significant likelihood of extended pain or suffering
- when successful treatment is more likely to bring extended unconsciousness or advanced dementia than cure or signif-icant amelioration
- when, whatever the medical condition, the available treat-

ments significantly increase the probability of a bad death, even if they also promise to extend life

I do not contend that the presumption to treat *must* change under those circumstances, only that it *may* and, ideally, *could* change. Great precision in making treatment decisions of this kind will not be possible. It is a matter of probabilities, of what is "likely" but not inevitable. There will always be a risk of making a mistake. My point is the need to balance risk, to see a poor, harsh death as a risk also, not simply death itself as *the* risk. The goal in shifting the presumption to treat is to enhance a quick, conscious, and socially engaged death, of a kind that is biologically plausible and the ordinary lot of other biological creatures. It is no less designed to minimize the chances of pain, of the suffering that comes from extended illness, and of the twilight or zombielike state that is the result of severe dementia or PVS. There is no good reason why a person who might have died quickly and easily in an earlier era should now have to die a worse death or remain alive much longer under degrading circumstances. Why should we have to accept this kind of medical "progress"?

Put another way, if earlier deaths from infectious disease had many of the characteristics of the peaceful death now desired, it is sensible and appropriate to seek to recapture as many of them as we can. Pneumonia and urinary tract disease, once common causes of death, are now all too routinely treated, even though they might allow a comparatively easy death. Their routine treatment allows the slow, destructive decline of the chronic and degenerative diseases to continue, bringing death by inches and reducing the possibility of a peaceful death. I do not underestimate the practical difficulties here. But the first and most important step in actual clinical practice is to change the presumption and the kinds of decisions it engenders, as much as the changed nature of the illnesses, that lead to poor deaths. Treating the prospect or even the possibility of a poor death as a significant reason to consider different treatment options, not just the conventional prospect of cure or disease amelioration, will in itself introduce an important change.

Care and caution are necessary in working toward this change. If it is carried out without the informed consent of a patient, it is a basic offense against that person's dignity. If the person desiring a shift in the presumption leaves in his wake undischarged social or familial obligations, a wrong could be done to others; the desire for a peaceful death does not override such obligations. If the presumption is too lightly changed, there could be a significant loss of the potential for still-unrealized personal development. That said, however, the basic point must be made: there can be no obligation to court a poor death, and every claim to want, and ask the assistance of medicine in providing, a peaceful death. This should be as much a part of the goals of medicine as the struggle with disease and illness. Until the advent of modern medicine, it always was.

Would these same considerations apply in making a decision to terminate treatment of an incompetent patient who had never expressed, before the onset of incompetence, a desire or preference? No. Much greater care would be in order, but that should not necessarily mean a maximum therapeutic effort. We can still ask which choice that we could make would best balance the need to respect the value of the person and the preservation of some level of health over against the value of not exposing that person to an undue risk of a bad death. We can see ourselves as protectors both of the life of the person and the possibility of a peaceful death. That may not be easy to carry out, but at least we know we owe the person, if at all possible, a peaceful death. That duty must be part of our reckoning.[3]

Stages of Treatment Termination

If the presumption to treat needs to be changed, how can that concretely be done? The most feasible way is to identify points where decisions to stop or abate life-extending treatment could be made, and to make use of them. We can turn technological brinkmanship on its head by choosing to stop treatment well short of the brink to which an aggressive technology can take us. Five different levels are candidates for such decisions.

Stage 1: A refusal to respond at all to health threats, even to seek diagnosis for medical symptoms or to engage in any kind of presymptomatic screening for the possible presence of disease; only palliative relief of symptoms sought. This is the most radical possibility, already embraced by some religious positions and frequently chosen by elderly patients who have decided they are ready to die. It is, in effect, a refusal to engage in any kind of relationship with therapeutic medicine. Common sense would, to be sure, accept the need for palliative relief of pain and discomfort as a fatal illness progressed, and perhaps even a minor therapeutic intervention solely to enhance the possibility of a peaceful death.

What are some important considerations in thinking about this possibility? Would I be evading some responsibilities to people who still depend upon me? Would I be turning my back on some still-unrealized valuable possibilities in my life? Would I, in some cases, be courting the likelihood that, by refusing medical examination of an emergent malady, I would pass up the chance of a simple, effective treatment? Could I actually increase the possibility of a poor death by ignoring early symptoms? How would I distinguish between a fear of medical treatment and a fear of death, by no means the same?

Stage 2: A refusal to go beyond diagnosis or identification of a potentially lethal disease to any curative response to the condition; palliative relief of symptoms only. This stage leaves open the potentially valuable possibility of diagnosis but, once it is in hand, is prepared to forgo the ordinary treatments that would follow. A person wants to know what is wrong with her, simply in order to know what to expect, but does not want to do anything to cure it.

The obvious problem here is that it would not be easy to have knowledge and yet not act upon it. Nor would it be easy to withstand the pressures of family and friends if they disagreed with our reasoning, particularly if the diagnosis revealed a con-dition that might successfully be treated.

Stage 3: A refusal to accept any medical treatment, for curative or ameliorative purposes, that does not promise a high probability of success and a minimum of unpleasant side-effects. In this stage, the burden of proof for going ahead with treatment is on the prob-ability of achieving a successful outcome if it is to be accepted. The presumption is against treatment, but can be overcome by favorable odds. This level will be most attractive to those who want to find a good balance between their desire for continued life and their goal of a peaceful death; they will not want to risk the latter for the sake of the former.

Doctors and families tend to be optimistic if at all possible when considering critical illness; none of us enjoys contemplating the worst possibilities. But this tendency means that it may be hard for the patient to determine the real likelihood of a good outcome, to sort out the expression of hope from solid medical judgment.

Stage 4: A willingness to accept any medical treatment that offers even a low probability of a successful outcome. The shift behind the change of attitude from stage 3 to stage 4 is profound. The presumption becomes one of accepting treatment unless the odds of a successful outcome are slight, but this is combined with a willingness to see treatment stopped if the odds drastically change in a negative direction. Stage 4 accepts a significant degree of technological brinkmanship, but is willing to seek a point just short of the brink to draw a line, aware of the hazards of going too far.

The danger here is evident: as we approach a technological brinkmanship, the dangers of a wild, poor death increase dra-matically. The patient must, in this case, have a solid and re-alistic idea of the nature of the gamble being undertaken, and what will happen if it goes wrong.

Stage 5: An eagerness to pursue any medical treatment with even the remotest possibility of success. This stage is caught in the expres-sion "Everything should be done." The bias in favor of treatment is total here, often combined with a willingness to tolerate almost any degree of pain, suffering, or reduced mental capacity. This is technological brinkmanship without restraint, aiming to go as far as medical aggressiveness will allow.

"If you can't stand the heat, get out of the kitchen," says the old political adage. It applies here as well. A person must realistically be willing to run the risk of outright disaster to choose this course, and it will be important for such a person to have a clear understanding of what in life is so attractive that it justifies risking a terrible death—a risk for himself but also for those who must care for him.

Implementing the Stages

No doubt an informal use of such a stage approach is already in effect. Almost everyone will be able to think of a friend or a family member who chose one stage or another. I have known people who just walked out of hospitals rather than have a life-saving operation, or refused to undergo diagnostic tests otherwise indicated by serious symptoms. Missing, as far as I know, is a more formal, deliberate use of the stages in medical practice. Stage 4 is ordinarily assumed to be the appropriate one for most patients, pursued without discussion, and most patients would themselves probably choose it. Yet, if a peaceful death is to become more common and accessible, then the first three stages will have to be more directly presented as choices to patients.[4] Patients should also, of course, be able to try a stage for a time and then move to a different one later. What I am saying here applies to both withholding and withdrawing treatment.

Yet to present the stages as patient choices will hardly be sufficient. Any patient who chooses one of the first three stages must be assured that adequate relief of pain will be available—and informed as well that a total rejection of all advanced therapies, ordinarily of a curative kind, could in some circumstances increase pain and suffering. Patient education will thus be crucial.

If patients are to choose to forgo treatment, especially relatively simple ones, they must know what to expect. It may be all too easy for the nervous patient, fearful of treatment, to choose one of the first three stages, not out of fear of a poor death, but out of a latent fear of the treatments that might sustain or extend life. Some people are more fearful of doctors and their treatments than of serious illness—a position that is not always rational.

Considerable skill on the part of physicians will be necessary to effect a more formal embracing of the stage approach I am suggesting. They will have to be willing to work with, and help, patients who deliberately refuse to choose treatments the physicians believe could benefit them. The physicians will themselves have to be willing to forgo the use of even simple therapies—inexpensive and painless antibiotics, for instance—that have been customary. They will have to inform themselves, so they can inform their patients, about the actual burden of pain and suffering a choice of one of the first three stages might carry with it. Patient ambivalence could be significant, particularly when patients are under family pressure (as will be common) to struggle against death. Families must come to understand that the choice of the means necessary for a peaceful death will require that they overcome some of their own reluctance. They must be helped to understand that a peaceful death is, if death has become inescapable, the most satisfying option for both patient and family. A peaceful death, when it can be achieved, is as much a benefit to a patient's family as to the patient.

Creating a Context for a Peaceful Death

To find a place within medicine, the goal of a peaceful death must, at the least, be understood as an integral part of medicine, an effort to bring death once again within its borders. This is best done by admitting the obvious, that every nonviolent death takes place as the result of an illness; illness and death cannot be separated, nor, more broadly, can aging, illness, and death be wholly separated. Illness could then be seen, not only as the enemy of life, but also as the necessary and inevitable means of death, to be accepted as much as death itself should be accepted. A change in the traditional presumption to treat—recognizing that its roots lie in technological brinkmanship and the confusion of the technological imperative and the sanctity of life—will help mightily in giving death a softer, more thoughtful place in medical practice. Becoming more conscious of the choice among different stages of termination of treatment will expand the options available to patients, now primarily restricted to an automatic expectation of aggressive treatment, to be stopped only when patently useless.

Yet none of this is likely to take place, or be understood as acceptable, apart from a supportive medical, cultural, and economic context. The law should not stand in the way of acceptable personal choice and decent medical practice, and the reforms of recent years have worked toward removing obstacles to choice. But, as I tried to show in an earlier chapter, it is naïve to look to legal reform alone to solve a problem with much deeper roots. Advance directives will fail to do all the good they might unless the rapidly changing medical technology that makes them so difficult to apply in practice can be better understood and domesticated. Families who are delegated the responsibility to make terminal decisions will not easily be able to discharge their duty unless they have a better grasp of the moral significance of terminating treatment, and, most important, recognize that their decision to stop treatment is not the same as killing.

Most needed for the future is a more comprehensive sense of the place of the understanding of death, and the care of the critically ill and dying, in two major contexts: in scientific medicine and medical practice, and in the economics of health care.

1. Scientific Medicine and Medical Practice. Contemporary scientific medicine has been fascinated by, and single-mindedly drawn to, forestalling death and reducing human mortality. As discussed earlier, the bias of research is to struggle against death, whereas the need of clinicians is to find a more satisfying way of accepting the death of their patients. There is only one serious way to resolve some of that tension: to reorient the goals of both scientific and clinical medicine away from an unbalanced bias toward cure and the reduction of mortality, and back toward a renewed emphasis on the ancient and original aim of care and comfort (which I mean also to encompass necessary nonmedical social services). It should be understood that caring is the most basic value in medicine, the one that should ordinarily take priority and that, in the end, is always indispensable. The same cannot be said of cure, which is not always needed.[5]

Why should there be a heightened emphasis on caring? One reason is the inevitability of death: cure will eventually run out for every patient, and only caring will be possible. No less important, in an era of chronic and degenerative disease, with the rising burden of those who cannot be cured, a different kind of medicine is needed: one that recognizes its own limits, that knows when it cannot effect a cure or can do so only at too high an economic or human price. It has been said, correctly enough, that the future belongs to chronic illness; in that case, the future of medicine should be oriented toward the care and treatment of such illnesses, many of which will end with death.

Most of us are likely to get sick from, and slowly die of, some disease that medicine cannot cure. We will need a medicine that accepts its own limitations, has put aside fantasies of medical miracles, has settled down to the enduringly important business of helping us live out, and die with, incurable illness. We will need the touch of human hands, decent long-term and home care, solid primary-care medicine, and those auxiliary social and economic supports that make life at least bearable.

Continued progress in medicine will and must be sought, but now with a sobered sense of its possibilities, perversities, and boundaries. Its possibilities are by no means inexpensive, and an unwise pursuit of them can jeopardize other important social needs. The perversities of progress should be no less apparent by now: the unintended consequences (e.g., longer life, greater illness), and the double-edged nature of some progress (e.g., rescuing a low-birth-weight baby, dooming it to a harsh life). The limits of progress are both financial (not everything can be afforded) and biological (old age and death can be manipulated, not conquered). The unwillingness of scientific medicine to accept death from disease, to believe that progress will allow the overcoming of fatal disease, must be changed. The idea of progress still will, and should, have its place. But medicine must ask just what kind of progress most contributes to the overall well-being of *mortal* creatures. A greater emphasis on quality of life rather than length of life, on the relief of pain and suffering, on understanding the origins of illness and working to modify their human impact, would all be ways of changing the agenda of scientific progress. As Leon R. Kass has written, it is "one more false goal of medicine . . . [to aim for] the prolongation of life, or the prevention of death. . . . On the contrary, medicine *should* be interested in preventing these [fatal] diseases or, failing that, in restoring their victims to as healthy a condition as possible. But it is precisely because they are causes of *unhealth,* and only secondarily because they are killers, that we should be interested in preventing or combating them."[6]

The future role of the doctor should come to reflect this kind of shift. A stronger place for family medicine and primary care is imperative—that is, for a first line of response to human mortality that puts a human face on medicine. What do we most need from medicine? We surely need it to keep us alive and to make us well, when it can do so. No less fundamentally, we need comfort and reassurance. The contemporary emphasis on technique and technology, scanting as it does the human dimensions of good medical care, fundamentally fails to comprehend human nature. That nature is able to accept death and understands, at least when pressed, that illness and aging are inescapable. But facing these circumstances generates anxiety, fear, a sense of loss and threat. Physicians need as much skill in dealing with those facets of human life as they do with the machines and drugs that can help the body.

Otherwise, medicine misses the point. What is that point? It is not the fact that we die that is intolerable, or at least not for medical reasons. What is intolerable is that medicine will not shape and order itself in a way that takes that fact seriously. This is the great source of anxiety in our present situation.

2. Economics and the Care of the Dying. There is a certain peculiarity in the economics of American health care that poses some serious threats to a peaceful death. It is the view that physicians owe it to patients to provide the most aggressive life-extending treatment, regardless of cost. Public-opinion polls have shown a public willingness to affirm the value of lifesaving treatment even at a tremendously high cost. Seventy-one percent of respondents to one survey said: "If it takes a million dollars to save a person, that should be spent."[7] The problem with this sentiment, otherwise admirable, is that it elevates the saving of life for its own sake to a level that is good neither for patient welfare nor for the economy. It thus tends to confirm the view that the saving of life is *the* purpose of medicine.

In a market economic system, moreover, where there are already profitable financial incentives in place to provide expensive lifesaving technologies, the combined force of money and morality can make it all the more difficult to find a way to a low-cost, nontechnological death. The latter is treated as a form of neglect, a profitless and anachronistic return to the ways of an era thought long passed. This general attitude creates a social context that powerfully reinforces the already present medical pressures that work against the goal of a peaceful death. The present economic system, in effect, blesses the wild death, the one that throws unlimited money and resources at death.

Nothing seems so much to disturb people as the idea that money, or the ability to pay, should stand in the way of lifesaving treatment. Human life, it is commonly said, is priceless; that belief reflects the great value attached to life in a culture with deep religious roots. Yet, of course, the daily reality of life in America, as well as in every other culture, requires economic limitations in all spheres, including lifesaving medicine. Even if there is no obvious shortage of money, no society allocates all of its resources to health care; and it is difficult to think of any developed society where, at least statistically, the investment of a few million dollars, or a few hundred million, could not save some additional lives—just as, we know, increasing the safety features on automobiles, or airplanes, or houses, could, at great expense, also save additional lives. The ordinary allocation of resources across a wide range of societal sectors—housing, education, welfare programs, defense, fire and police protection, and so on—means that money is, and must be, diverted from health care.

I cite these obvious facts to distinguish two situations, sometimes confused. One of them, just mentioned, is that no culture can allow health care to pre-empt all other societal needs totally. It cannot turn itself into a large hospital. This means that, however indirectly, some lives are lost that might otherwise be saved if *all* resources were devoted to health care. The other situation occurs when, consciously and directly, a decision is made to deny lifesaving care merely in order to save money, typically on the grounds that the expenditure is "not worth it." This kind of denial of care is most feared, for here it seems that human life is being given a price tag and, if its cost is too high, not protected by medicine from death. If the former situation is inevitable in any and all societies, however affluent—not all money can go to health care—the latter seems both unacceptable and avoidable.

Yet the growing costs of health care, particularly those of caring for an aging society in the company of ever more expensive technological medicine, are tending to bring the two situations together. The technological advances raise, in a stark and direct way, the question of whether they can be applied to all patients— or whether, if they are applied to all patients threatened with death, they will take money away from other medical conditions that are important but not life-threatening.

There is no doubt that we could, as a society, afford the level of technology available twenty or thirty years ago. But developments in contemporary technology, constant and steady, have made medicine much more costly per capita than it used to be. Bypass surgery for those in their eighties, or neonatal care running into the hundreds of thousands of dollars, represents a new problem for both ethics and economics. I would phrase the issue this way: even if we agree that everyone should have access to a decent level of health care, does this commit us to accepting whatever level of technological progress medical science brings, at whatever cost that may entail?

I do not see how this can be either affordable or defensible. Some limits must be set, limits that may make it perfectly clear in advance just who will not receive potentially lifesaving treatment. Yet the real question here is not the denial of health care as such, but the denial of some of the endless fruits of medical progress. If we now think it appropriate to offer bypass surgery for an octogenarian whose life may thus be saved, will we be equally obliged to offer an artificial heart to a nonogenarian when (as is certainly likely) that also becomes available? If the only test of economic acceptability is the efficacy of the treatment— if it works, that is, we should pay for it—then medical progress could well bankrupt us, or, more subtly, lead us to spend more on the health-care sector of the economy than on other sectors of great civic and social importance.

How can this situation be avoided? A start could be made by working toward a health-care system that has consensually and democratically developed a clear set of priorities, beginning first with a decision about how much to spend on health care as a general social expenditure. A health-care system that began with decent caring and social services for the sick, then guaranteed good pediatric and maternal care, general public-health measures, and primary and emergency medical care would, I believe, have the most defensible and economically sound priorities, those most likely to ensure a decent common level of health. Thereafter, with whatever funds remained (which would be significant), expensive technological medicine could be pursued, the form of medicine that has great benefits for some or even many individuals (kidney dialysis and organ transplantation, for example), but does not greatly improve overall societal health.

A clear priority system would recognize the need for some economic limits, thereby forcing a society to determine its most important needs and, when limits must be set, to do so in a way that does not select out some individuals as not "worth it." If, for example, a society decided it could not afford to follow medical progress to artificial hearts for those over age ninety, it would not be because those of such age are disvalued, but because of a priority system that assumed the first task of a health-care system to be helping the young to become old, not seeking ever-longer life through medical progress for those who have already become old.

The trouble with an open-ended system, of the kind existing in the United States, is not only that it admits of no natural boundaries to health expenditures, but also that it in effect refuses to accept death. Treating each and every death as an equal threat to the human good, equally to be resisted, creates two harms. One of them is the expenditure of a disproportionate amount of money on a comparatively few conditions, those that turn out to be amenable to expensive technological interventions. The other is the expenditure of a disproportionate amount of money at the fringes of life, working to save lives where the costs are high and the results, if good at all, marginal and short-term. In both cases—ironically, given the alleged dedication to life— money is diverted from health care for the many to serve the needs of the few. Only a society unduly fearful of death, and unduly captured by the notion that an unlimited amount of money should be spent on individual cases even at the neglect of public health, could end up with such a strange set of priorities.

Medical Futility

The general orientation and resource-allocation priorities of the health-care system can make a considerable difference, albeit indirectly for the most part, in the care of the dying. Of more direct and immediate impact will be the aggregate effect of what clinicians at the bedside come to consider futile or marginally useful treatment. As a concept, "futility" has both medical and moral dimensions.[8] Its medical feature is the probability that a particular treatment for a particular person will not be efficacious—that is, will not return the patient to good health or sustain the patient in any medically viable way. The moral feature is a judgment that some forms of medical treatment, with either a low or no probability of success, should be judged morally to be useless. If the two concepts are put together, a judgment of medical futility is medical insofar as it relies on judgments of probability of medical outcome, and moral to the extent that it relies upon judgments about whether the pursuit of low-probability outcomes is morally required.

There is already considerable pressure from physicians to be allowed to make judgments of medical futility themselves, without having to ask patients or their families. Their goal is not to avoid a doctor-patient interaction, but to be spared the pressure of unrealistic patient demands. It is one thing, they say, to be asked by a patient or his family to stop treatment; that is acceptable. It is still another to be asked to provide treatment of a kind they think futile or useless; that they take to be unacceptable, a threat to their professional integrity.

Their instinct is correct and reasonable here. Physicians ought not to be required to perform procedures, or provide treatment, that they believe will do no good. Yet we must protect the rights of patients to be informed of their situation; it would be arbitrary to allow physicians unilaterally to make those judgments. It would be better if the standards for doing so were established collectively, by joint bodies of laypeople and physicians. This might best be done in individual hospitals, where joint medical-lay panels could help establish an institutional policy sensitive to local needs and values. It should not, I believe, be done with individual patients on a case-by-case basis. Judgments of futility could then be made, and treatments denied, but on the basis of consensual norms and publicly visible policies.[9] The development of such policies would, of course, have a potentially significant impact on the options available to patients who choose stages 4 and 5 as outlined above. Some general societal standards would come to replace unlimited patient choice.

What would be the pertinence of such a development for the termination of treatment? It would be valuable if, in coming years, a consensus was achieved about futile treatment. "Futility" needs, however, to be understood in two senses: futile because no benefit whatever can be achieved from treatment, and futile because, given resource limitations, the treatment is economically unjustifiable within the available resources. Thus we must have a general social agreement on PVS and the right of physicians to withhold medical treatment to patients suffering from it, and an agreement on the forms of medical treatment that would be considered futile for those faced with imminent death from an acute or chronic illness, or from the slow death of dementia.

A standard of futility compatible with the goal of avoiding an unnecessarily painful or extended death would be particularly valuable. The test of futility could be twofold: first, an inability to arrest more than momentarily (a few days or weeks) a downward, deteriorating course; and, second, the probability, should that kind of effort be made, that a peaceful death would become increasingly unlikely. At that point, curative medical treatment has indeed become futile, and ought to be stopped. The standard is thus one that looks to the possibility of sustaining life in some decent fashion, but also, and simultaneously, to the choices necessary to enhance the possibility of a peaceful death.

The most difficult problem of futility judgments, and one that is impending, is whether to embody them in public policy. As matters now stand, it is customary for both federal and private health-care plans to provide reimbursement for the care of those in a PVS, paying the families and medical staffs that want treatment continued. Should financial support continue in the future? I believe that, in principle, it should not. Ideally speaking, it makes no sense, in light of budget restraints or humane public policy, to sustain with medical technology for an extended period the life of someone who will almost certainly never return to consciousness.

The temptation here is to adopt an either/or approach. If we consider the patient alive, then we must provide the patient with all those forms of health care that we would provide any other live person; or we may simply consider the patient as dead, even if not legally so, and stop all care. The problem, however, is that we as a society remain uncertain about the status of patients who manage to combine, in a bewildering way, elements both of life and death. An appropriate compromise, I believe, would be to provide minimal nursing care only, but not the extended artificially provided nutrition and hydration that many institutions now routinely provide (probably because of public disagreement about the moral status of someone in that condition).

My guess is that increasingly few people will believe for long that this form of "life" merits being called human. It is a moribund life sustained by technological artifact in the face of a biological condition crying out to come to an end, as it would ordinarily in nature. Yet, as long as disagreement persists, it would be unwise to stop treatment precipitately or high-handedly. That could seem to bespeak an indifference to the important convictions of some people, convictions not without some merit. But every effort should slowly be made to change those convictions and thus forge a social consensus that would form the basis of a new policy, which would refuse reimbursement for patients in that condition. A softer, perhaps more tolerable, alternative would be to assign a low priority to such treatment, to help assure it would not capture resources that could be better spent on more needy patients with a great chance of real recovery or amelioration of their condition.

A peaceful death should have both an individual and a public face. It can bring life to a fitting close for the individual, who is still connected to himself, by virtue of reason and self-consciousness, and to others, by virtue of being still within the circle of human companionship and caring. But death should also have a peaceful public face. The control and management of death, understood as an unavoidable part of life, should not consume an undue share of resources, as if the staying of death represented society's most important goal. People should have a chance to live a healthy life, avoid premature death, and then die without the ministrations of technological brinkmanship, which knows no boundaries in the war against mortality.

I would define a peaceful death in a public context as a death that, on the one hand, did not require a disproportionate share of resources for fighting illness and death, a practice that leads to economic violence, threatening other societal goods such as education and housing; and, on the other, rejected euthanasia and assisted suicide as still other forms of violence, though medical and social rather than economic.

What about family burdens as a form of quasi-domestic violence? It is not improper for people to worry about being a burden on their families or to wish they could spare them undue emotional or financial hardship. We can readily recognize the possibility of taking down with us, in a parallel destruction, those family members whose devotion—economic or emotional or both—is pressed too far. It is hard to see how a death that impoverishes a family, or destroys the later years of an elderly spouse, or wrecks the family life of a dutiful child caring for an elderly parent, can be called entirely peaceful in its broader ramifications.

At the same time, however, it is right and proper that we bear one another's illness and dying. We should not only be willing to care for others; no less important, we should allow them to care for us if there is no moral or humane way to avoid that burden. We do not need a medical system, and a set of moral values, that will impose upon families the drain of extended illness and death. We should be willing to bear what nature, and human mortality, bring to us. But there is no reason why we should have to bear technologically extended deaths. A family member should reject them for the sake of the family's welfare after he or she is gone. And family members should, when a patient is incompetent and death on the way, not be forced, through guilt or a confusion about killing and allowing to die, to believe that a termination of treatment is wrongful killing. It is not. It is not killing at all.

Chapter 7

WATCHING AND WAITING

Although I did not understand it then, when my longtime friend asked me to visit him at his farm during my summer vacation his purpose was almost surely to pull together the strands of our relationship over the years and, without directly letting me know it, to say goodbye. I had not seen him for a few years, and his altered appearance was unsettling—a thin and wasted body, and a face that showed pain as his constant companion. He looked older than his seventy years. We talked, but not about his illness, much less his coming death. When I tried to do that, he changed the subject—not by way of evasion, I came to realize, but out of a fear felt by many who have been ill a long time, that they will seem caught in self-pity, soon wearing out our solicitude.

We talked instead the way we had always talked, about what we were thinking and feeling and about our plans for the future. He was, I could see in retrospect, vague about his plans. A few months later, he died; his was the kind of death I have been working to understand and describe in this book. As his wife wrote afterward, "On the day that turned out to be his last, he told us it was time to die, asked us not to prolong his life but to let him go. We sent him along with aching love and blessing on his journey, and he left us, quietly and peacefully—as beautiful and noble and spiritual in death as he was in life."

How could someone in such pain die that way, I had to ask myself? A more general question also came to mind. What, I wondered, have been the common traits of those people whose peaceful deaths I have seen or heard about? One point stands out: their peaceful death did not seem a matter of good fortune only. They did not die differently from the way they had lived. It was as if they gathered into one culminating moment all those personal traits and virtues that had served them well in life. Some were in pain and some were not. In some cases their death was premature, in some cases not. What mattered in each case, as far as I could see, was what they made of their situation.

They did not treat their dying as bad luck, but simply the way things were. They accepted their death, bowing without complaint to its coming, some for religious reasons and some for reasons of other kinds. They did not think a loss of control of their bodies and their lives meant a loss of dignity and self-respect. If they required a bedpan and the humiliation of a public display of their wastes, they just put up with that. If there was pain, they endured it. If there was sorrow, they did not pour it on themselves. They grieved for those who would have to bear their loss. They sought to put those around them at ease, anxious not to carry others down with them. They took their leave, making it a point to see their friends, even if they did not always say why. They were conscious and lucid almost until the end, in part because they had asked that their medical treatment be stopped earlier than it might have been.

Most of all, I sensed, they put death in its place, downplaying its importance and drama. They saw that it would be a greater blow to others than to themselves. They had reconciled themselves to their end but knew this would be harder for others. One of the great harms done by the modern, and particularly medical, ambivalence about death has been to magnify its damage and significance in our lives, creating excess fear and uncertainty.

Those who die peacefully seem to have understood that, and thus sought to find ways to make death less, not more, important. This may have been a skill that other generations mastered better than ours, even if, lacking much choice, they were driven to it by necessity. But ours is still the same necessity, just dressed up in fine clothes to disguise the underlying reality. Those who die peacefully seem to find ways to throw off those garments, and see death for what it is, our fate.

Was there no luck in all of this? Of course. They could have had a condition that choked them to death. Or brought them to unconsciousness long before they died. Or financially ruined their families. People die that way, even though, we may rightly remind ourselves, the odds are against it. Yet, because they had been the kind of people who accepted the good and bad in life, I suspect they might well have endured more terrible deaths with the same grace. I suppose they were lucky in having a circle of family and friends who remained with them all the way, who visited and talked and watched. But was that really chance? They had always been the kind of people who drew others to them, in bad times as well as good.

As I tried to think about these deaths, however, something else occurred to me. I cannot say for certain that they were not suffering; possibly, beneath the surface, were fear, dread, anxiety, and perhaps even more pain than we thought. Yet I came to see why I would never know the truth about this. They were the kind of people who had always known when to hold their tongue, to conceal their pain, understanding full well that such a discipline is part of a tolerable life with others, both the living and the dying parts of it. If their deaths were, from the inside, far more terrible than I could know, they hid this well, and thereby made it easier for those of us who survived to face our own deaths better.

I recount these observations to make two points. The first is simply to articulate a perception I find both reassuring and terrifying: we must find our own meaning for death and die our own deaths. I find it reassuring to know that the kind of person

I am can and will make a difference in the way I die, in my capacity to adapt and endure. I can see, by the living and dying of others, the truth of that perception. I need not be a mere victim, whatever my dying may have in store for me. I also find it terrifying to know that I should even now, with death not immediately in sight, be working to become that kind of person, and the sooner the better. I am fearful that I may fail, or may have the kind of bad luck that would overwhelm even someone otherwise ready for, and able to accept, death. I know the kind of person I would like to become, but I have no assurance I will succeed. That is the task before me, with the outcome in doubt until I am put to the test.

My second point is this: we cannot, or are unlikely to, find a meaning in death entirely on our own, even if this seems the demand placed upon us. We can scarcely hope to find on our own the answer to a question that has troubled and puzzled the human species for thousands of years. We need the help of others, of a community whose meaning we can share, making it our own with the same strength as if we had discovered it for ourselves. My second point, therefore, seems to contradict my first. We must find our own meaning in death, and yet we cannot easily, if at all, do it alone. Is there a way out of this dilemma? I am not certain, and it will have to be left as an open question, the answer to which will make a great difference in the years to come. I will try to offer some suggestions of a possible direction in which to look.

Looking for Meaning

Why do I say we cannot find our own meaning? By "meaning," first of all, I comprehend especially the notion of coherence and explanation. Actions or events will have meaning for us if they make a kind of sense: they are coherent with other things in life that we already understand, and we can see how they came about, even if not fully. Not everything that has meaning need be acceptable. I might come to understand the biological inevitability of death without thereby accepting the natural order that made it inevitable. My death, that is, can make sense even if I find that sense intolerable. At least I can understand what is happening. It is even better, to be sure, if I can find some justification for the way things are, but that may not be possible.

By "meaning" I also want to convey, however, the way we as human beings create communities of meaning. Words have meanings for us because we have come, as people living and talking together, to share through language and symbols our understanding of things, the external objects and events in the world and the internal feelings, thoughts, and yearnings within ourselves. The great events of life and death come to have a meaning, I believe, in a similar way. We make of them symbols of good or evil, order or chaos, threat or reassurance, and, equally, we make of them patterns of order and explanation. We learn how to talk and think about them. We have come to understand birth, for instance, not simply as a particular biological phenomenon, the way we all come into the world, but also as a social event. It is the way we renew the species, create our families, and bring into the world new possibilities.

We can smile with pleasure at the sound of a newborn child because that sound betokens renewal, hope, rejuvenation, continuance into the future. We come to feel part of a community because we find its system of symbols, of interpretation, and of meaning plausible and satisfying; and we know how to share with others the language of that community. We can, therefore, talk with others about the joy that the newborn child brings and understand the place that the new life, and the meaning it carries, fits into our understanding of the order of things. So too, when we encounter on occasion someone for whom a new child is a burden, a threat to some other sense of order, we can understand how a birth can have a very different, threatening, meaning.

Yet it is precisely when we try to discover the meaning death has in our society that we run into trouble. It is not there to be found, at least not in our common life together, by which I mean to encompass our relationships with strangers as well as intimates. There is, in that fuller sense, no common response to death, no shared ritual, no clear conventions of succor, sorrow, and grief. They may be found, but not necessarily, within particular religious and ethnic groups, at least for those members who have remained close to their traditions and rituals. But increasingly, I suspect, the emptiness about death that marks our common life infects even those groups, if only because they cannot easily remain isolated. Here we come to what may be our most important deficit: we do not have the shared sense of destiny that Philippe Ariès identified as central to the possibility of a tame death in an earlier time. We have tried, to be sure, to find substitutes, but in each case they turn out to be ways of better mastering and controlling death, not of finding a common way to seek and share its meaning and accept its inevitability.

It is worth recollecting what those substitutes have been. The first, and still the most fateful, was to make of death a medical problem, a matter of understanding the diseases and pathologies that kill human bodies and then taking arms against them. The religious or philosophical meaning of death was pushed aside as a question. In its place was put the scientific effort to understand the causes of death. Science could thus pick up most triumphantly on an ancient theme, that of death as an accident, the result of trivial incidents or choices, each of which could have been otherwise.[1] Medical science could in its own way agree with the plaintive lament of Simone de Beauvoir: "There is no such thing as a natural death: nothing that ever happens to a man is ever natural, since his presence calls the world into question. All men must die: but for every man his death is an accident, and, even if he knows it and consents to it, an unjustifiable violation."[2] To this sense of violation, science had a response: get rid of the causes of death, *écrasez l'infâme.*

Yet death continued to exist despite the scientific wars against it, its timing and circumstances changed but not its final and still-dominating reality. Now what was to be done? The answer was soon forthcoming and is still in the process of refinement.

Why not just put death out of sight, take the sick bodies out of houses and put them in hospitals, and take the dead bodies out of living rooms and put them in funeral parlors. As the historian James J. Farrell nicely reminds us: "The middle-class funeral reformers promoted death control as a fight against the fear of death. In the fight, they attempted to assassinate both fear and death. . . . By redefining death, they spared many people from an incapacitating fear of death, and from the public expression of their private emotions. By assigning the care of the body to specialists, they liberated people from death's bodily gruesomeness. By securing the ritual of the funeral in a web of social conventions under the supervision of a funeral director, they allowed bereaved people to pay their final respects with a minimum of pain and involvement. By curtailing the lengthy formality of mourning customs, they prevented death from overshadowing the lives of relatives and friends of the deceased. Motivated by an obsession for order and by a humane compassion for suffering people, funeral directors met with some success in controlling the effects of death."[3]

But not enough success. For all their skills—now extended to that even more distancing ceremony, the memorial service—the funeral directors have no control over the dying that brings people to them. If medicine has failed to control death, and funeral ceremonies cannot altogether manage the way people feel and think about death—cannot, that is, take away the anxiety its prospect inspires—there was still one other maneuver to be tried. That move, of course, is our present emphasis upon rights and choices: empower people to sign documents specifying how they want to die, to appoint surrogates to speak in their behalf, and in that way death will be pacified.

Such a tactic is not going to work either, though surely it will have some benefits. But, then, medical science and the funeral industry have provided us some benefits also. Just not enough, never enough, and, even worse, giving us more than a hint that we may be even worse off in dealing with death than we were in supposedly more primitive, backward, and innocent times.

We looked to science, that great modern faith, for relief, and then to the art of psychological management as skillfully deployed by grief therapists and funeral directors, and then, as a last hope, to law and regulation. For all that, we still lack the foundation for a peaceful death—a foundation that can only be of one kind, a shared communal meaning of death, one that has some depth and richness. Without that, the other measures will continue to fail, and the nakedness of their evasions will stand out even more.

Death and Solidarity

By such a shared meaning I have in mind not necessarily a precisely agreed-upon common interpretation of death. Instead, I mean some agreement on what it is we need to think together about, and how we ought to express together the communal solidarity that is broken by death, best expressed by public symbols and open grieving. The test is not the death of my known neighbor or family member but of the stranger. We need to see that these deaths matter to us as well.

To say we need a "shared communal meaning" is to deny the sufficiency of membership in a religious or ethnic group that itself offers an interpretation of death and a way of understanding it. That is surely helpful, and there is no doubt that many people die, and well, with the embrace of a particular community, usually religious. But it is increasingly hard in modern society to live only in such communities, probably impossible. We need something more general, for all of us together, not only so that the smaller religious communities will not be entirely bereft of some larger societal support, but also so that those without the benefit of such communities will not be left empty-handed at the time of their dying. Because of our increasingly extended old age, there is a good chance that many of us will die in the company of strangers, our spouses and friends dead before us, and perhaps even our children. We would do well to hope those strangers will have a sensitivity to death, that they will know how to talk with and to comfort us, and that they will see in our dying their own eventual fate and thus our common lot.

Where can that shared meaning be found? I stumble at this point. I do not know with any certainty. I only know that it is one of the great and necessary cultural tasks before us, just as important as the more generally accepted need to find some shared way of understanding the human relationship to nature, to deal with our environmental problems. I can only offer some suggestive pointers, working outward from some insights already part of our common patrimony.

We might well begin by speculating that a sense of common meaning may be more of a mosaic of elements than some single, decisive insight. I have suggested that it must encompass at least a view of the self and a picture of nature. We surely need before death to reconsider the self and the way it situates itself. A self obsessed with control—either to remedy the failures of medicine to give us a biological domination of death, or to express a commitment to the value of self-determination—will be a deficient and defective self, less flexible and protean in the face of mortality than it ought to be. A self that is, by contrast, willing to bend and shape itself to the contours of mortality—sometimes harsh and demanding, if we are unfortunate, sometimes kindly and forgiving, if we are lucky—will be better able to meet the demands of death.

We need no less to reconsider the place of nature, and particularly the human relationship to nature, to find the line between human actions leading to death, and the independent actions of nature. Nature has not been banished, and it is one of the more egregious of contemporary conceits to think it has been. A consideration of nature leads directly to medicine, which attempts to understand and control nature in the name of health and the preservation of life.

At its best, however, medicine can only work within the boundaries of nature, moving the furniture and fittings of our mortality about with some great skill, but never changing the inexorability of that mortality. A medicine that embodied an acceptance of death within it would represent a great change in the common conception of medicine, and might then set the stage for seeing the care of the dying not as an afterthought when all else has failed but as itself one of the ends of medicine. The goal of a peaceful death should be as much a part of the purpose of medicine as that of the promotion of good health. That means medicine must abandon the modern cultic myth that in the cure of disease lies the cure of death. All good health eventually comes to an end, and nowhere is our human fragility more manifest than when we are fit and healthy. It cannot, and will not, last. Disease and death will have their day.

If those parts of the mosaic of the meaning of death could be put in place, a start would have been made. But that would still not be enough. "Why do I have to die?" William Paley, the founder of CBS and a man used to power and control and glamour, supposedly asked on his deathbed. No answer was forthcoming, of course. It is an awkward question to put before the public, yet also an arresting one, which is no doubt why the media underscored it in the story of Mr. Paley's death. It is the question to which we all want an answer, and the question we find most difficult to talk with one another about. Yet all we have left now is the need to find a way to talk together as people about death. We need to see whether a civic conversation can be developed that would blend the insights of the great religions of the world—for they have animated particular communities over the century, providing a road map for them—and our secular understanding of philosophy and human biology. What should we talk about? There are two directions our conversation can take—not necessarily the only directions, but I believe the most fruitful.

One of them expresses the great profundity and contradiction at the heart of human life: that death itself is necessary for life, and that life cannot be understood without seeing the place, and the necessary place, of death. The other direction seeks, even if it does not find, some transcendence. The theologian John

Bowker captures well the first direction when, concluding his exploration of the meanings of death in the great world religions, he writes: "The religious affirmation of value *includes* the reality of death, maybe as the last enemy, but also as the necessary condition of life. Attempts to evade death, or to pretend that it is not serious, or to deny its necessary place in the ordering of life, have almost always been regarded by the major religious traditions as false or dangerous or subversive of truth."[4]

In the idea of sacrifice, Bowker sees religion and science coming together. Science makes clear to us that death is a necessary condition of life. Can we, he asks, have human life on any other terms than death? Can my children's children live unless I die? For science, he argues persuasively, the answer is as "equally emphatic" as it is in religion—no. The continuation of biological life in general requires in particular the death of each and every creature that appears. We are as individuals the living sacrifices that human existence as such requires, our own as well as every other form of life. Here, then, we can see why, in a certain view of religion and science, death is and must always remain both friend and enemy, as much the one as the other.

This is a hard truth to accept. It offers us no easy way out. But it does offer us reason to bear with one another, and bear one another, in working through the ways and cycles of nature. It requires of us a view of the human condition broader than that of our own fate and gives us a common stake in the ongoing enterprise of human life—even if, inescapably, that enterprise must grind us down as individuals.

Some will feel that is not enough, though for now it seems enough for me. I wish there could be more, a better direction. For some there will be: out of the struggle, the sacrifice, the suffering, there will be individual redemption and the possibility of transcendence. I can envy those who have such hope, even if I cannot share it. This is the bent of the great Western religions, and it is only the superstitions of modernism that would, with the back of the hand, dismiss that possibility.

We hate death, I believe, because it means the end of the life that has given us what we have, and what we can become. We no less hate death because it is the final, the crowning, reminder once and for all that we are finite, bounded creatures. We see death at the end of the road in our lives, but it is forever fore-shadowed in living our daily lives. We cannot have everything we want in life. We cannot have our dreams live on forever, even if we can achieve them for a time. We cannot stop things from going wrong, however much we dedicate ourselves to con-trol. Could we bear death better if life were perfect? Probably not. The pain of separation from life would be all the greater. It is our human condition that is the problem, of which death is the great token. But only the token.

Can death, and the life in which it is embedded, be tran-scended? I do not see this for myself, but I hope to live the remainder of my days in a way that at least puts me in a position to be (as Wordsworth put it) "surprised by joy." It is unlikely but perhaps not impossible. I wait and watch.

NOTES

Introduction: Can Death Be Shaped to Our Own Ends?

1. Nathaniel Hawthorne, *Our Old Home*, quoted in D. J. Enright, ed., *The Oxford Book of Death* (New York: Oxford University Press, 1987), p. 319.
2. M. Powell Lawton, Miriam Ross, and Allen Glicksman, "The Quality of the Last Year of Life of Older Persons," *Milbank Quarterly*, vol. 68, no. 1 (1990), pp. 1–28; Dwight B. Brock, Daniel J. Foley, and Katalin Losonczy, "A Survey of the Last Days of Life: Overview and Initial Results," *Proceedings of the American Statistical Association, Social Statistics Section*, 1987, pp. 306–11; Harold R. Leutzner et al., "The Quality of Life in the Year Before Death," *American Journal of Public Health*, vol. 82, no. 8 (August 1992), pp. 1092–98.
3. See, in particular, Robert M. Veatch, *Death, Dying and the Biological Revolution*, rev. ed. (New Haven, Conn.: Yale University Press, 1989); Robert F. Weir, *Abating Treatment with Critically Ill Patients* (New York: Oxford University Press, 1989); Robert W. Wennberg, *Terminal Choices: Euthanasia, Suicide, and the Right to Die* (Grand Rapids, Mich.: William B. Eerdmans, 1989); President's Commission for the Study of Ethical Problems in Medicine and Biomedical and Behavioral Research, *Deciding to Forego Life-Sustaining Treatment* (Washington, D.C.: U.S. Government Printing Office, 1983); Dennis J. Horan and David Mall, eds., *Death, Dying and Euthanasia* (Frederick, Md.: University Publications of America, 1980).

Chapter 1: The First Illusion: Mastering Our Medical Choices

1. An interesting Gallup Poll, published in early 1991, found that "Americans not only don't appear to think about death, they don't worry about it either," and presented data to show that only 23 percent of those surveyed said they feared death (George Gallup and Frank Newport, "Mirror of America: Fear of Dying," *Gallup Poll News Service*, vol. 55, no. 3 [January 6, 1991], p. 1). This study shows the importance of distinguishing between a fear of death—that is, being dead—and the process of dying, which I believe elicits far greater fear. Even with the Gallup findings, however, some caution is in order. To what extent have those who fear death repressed that fear? There can be no good answer to this question, but it would be remarkable if contemporary Americans have found some secret solution to the age-old human fear of death.

2. William Butler Yeats, "Sailing to Byzantium," in Richard J. Finneran, ed., *W. B. Yeats: The Poems* (New York: Macmillan, 1983), p. 193. The full quotation is: "An aged man is but a paltry thing, / A tattered coat upon a stick. . . ."

3. Philippe Ariès, *The Hour of Our Death*, trans. Helen Weaver (New York: Alfred A. Knopf, 1981), pp. 5–28; see also Philippe Ariès, *Western Attitudes Toward Death*, trans. Patricia M. Ranum (Baltimore: Johns Hopkins University Press, 1974).

4. Ariès, *Hour of Our Death*, p. 28.

5. Ibid., p. 5.

6. Ibid., p. 6.

7. Alexander Solzhenitsyn, *Cancer Ward* (New York: Farrar, Straus and Giroux, 1969), pp. 96–97, quoted in Ariès, *Western Attitudes*, p. 13.

8. Quoted in Ken Burns, *The Civil War: An Illustrated History* (New York: Alfred A. Knopf, 1990), p. 300.

9. Ben Jonson, "An Elegy on the Lady Jane Paulet," in D. J. Enright, ed., *The Oxford Book of Death* (New York: Oxford University Press, 1987), p. 67.

10. Ariès, *Hour of Our Death*, p. 11.

11. Ibid., pp. 559, 603, 604.

12. The general resistance to, or outright rejection of, Ariès's thesis

that death was once tame has not been shared by historians passing
professional judgment upon his work. See, for instance, Rudolph
M. Bell's review of *The Hour of Our Death*, in *Journal of Modern
History*, vol. 55 (June 1983), pp. 298–300; Judith Modell, review
in *Journal of Interdisciplinary History*, vol. 13 (Winter 1983), pp.
544–46; Terence Des Pres, review in *Yale Review*, vol. 71, no. 2
(January 1982), pp. 241–93.

13. Ariès, *Hour of Our Death*, p. 604.
14. Ariès, *Western Attitudes*, p. 28.
15. Ariès, *Hour of Our Death*, p. 605.
16. Ibid., pp. 612, 614.
17. Ernest Becker, *The Denial of Death* (New York: Free Press, 1973);
    Geoffrey Gorer, "The Pornography of Death," *Encounter*, vol. 5
    (October 1955), pp. 49–52.
18. William James, *Varieties of Religious Experience: A Study in Human
    Nature* (New York: Mentor, 1958), p. 281, quoted in Becker,
    Denial of Death, p. 16.
19. Quoted: Ariès, *Hour of Our Death*, p. 516.
20. Ibid., p. 595.
21. Ibid., p. 614.
22. Ibid.
23. Ariès, *Western Attitudes*, p. 106.
24. Ibid., p. 107.
25. A thorough and informative discussion of advance directives can
    be found in chapters 10–12 of Alan Meisel, *The Right to Die* (New
    York: John Wiley & Sons, 1989), pp. 311–428.
26. See especially Coordinating Council on Life-Sustaining Medical
    Treatment Decision Making by the Courts, *Guidelines for State
    Court Decision Making in Authorizing or Withholding Life-Sustaining
    Medical Treatment* (Williamsburg, Va.: National Center for State
    Courts, 1991); see also Pat Milmore McCarrick, "Living Wills and
    Durable Power of Attorney: Advance Directive Legislation and
    Issues," *Scope Note* 2 (Washington, D.C.: National Reference Cen-
    ter for Bioethics Literature, Georgetown University, 1991), pp.
    1–20; see also The Hastings Center, *Guidelines on the Termination
    of Life-Sustaining Treatment and the Care of the Dying* (Briarcliff
    Manor, N.Y.: The Hastings Center, 1987).
27. Cicely Saunders, Dorothy H. Summers, Neville Teller, eds., *Hos-
    pice: The Living Idea* (London: Edward Arnold, 1981); Saudol

Stoddard, *The Hospice Movement* (New York: Random House, 1978).

28. Alan C. Mermann et al., "Learning to Care for the Dying: A Survey of Medical Schools and a Model Course," *Academic Medicine*, vol. 66, no. 1 (January 1991), pp. 35–38.

29. See especially Marion Danis et al., "A Prospective Study of Advance Directives for Life-Sustaining Care," *New England Journal of Medicine*, vol. 324, no. 13 (March 28, 1991), pp. 882–95; see also George J. Annas, "The Health Care Proxy and the Living Will," *New England Journal of Medicine*, vol. 324, no. 17 (April 25, 1991), pp. 1210–13.

30. I am indebted to Marsha Zandbergen, director of membership services, National Hospice Organization, Arlington, Va., for this information. I want to emphasize the great value of the hospice movement, whose methods should be much more widely used.

31. See Robert J. Blendon, Ulrike S. Szalay, and Richard A. Knox, "Should Physicians Aid Their Patients in Dying: The Public Perspective," *Journal of the American Medical Association*, vol. 267, no. 19 (May 20, 1992), pp. 2658–62.

32. Lawrence J. Schneiderman et al., "Effects of Offering Advance Directives on Medical Treatment Goals and Costs," *Annals of Internal Medicine* vol. 117 (October 1, 1992), pp. 599–606; Ashwini Sehgal et al., "How Strictly Do Dialysis Patients Want Their Advance Directives Followed?," *Journal of the American Medical Association*, vol. 267, no. 1 (January 1, 1992), pp. 59–63; see also Joan M. Teno et al., "Impact of Advance Directives on Decision Making," *The Gerontologist*, vol. 31 (1991), p. 41; Joanne Lynn, "Why I Don't Have a Living Will," *Law, Medicine & Health Care*, vol. 19, nos. 1–2 (Summer 1991), pp. 101–4; Marshall B. Kapp, "State Statutes Limiting Advance Directives: Death Warrants or Life Sentences?" *Journal of the American Geriatric Society*, vol. 40 (1992), pp. 722–26.

33. James C. Riley, *Sickness, Recovery and Death* (Iowa City: University of Iowa Press, 1989), p. 109; see also Arthur E. Imhof, "From the Old Mortality Pattern to the New: Implications of a Radical Change from the Sixteenth to the Twentieth Century," *Bulletin of the History of Medicine*, vol. 59, no. 1 (Spring 1985), pp. 1–29; James C. Riley, "The Risk of Being Sick: Morbidity Trends in Four Countries," *Population and Development Review*, vol. 16, no.

3 (September 1990), pp. 403–31. See also Jack Larkin, *The Reshaping of Everyday Life* (New York: Harper & Row, 1988), especially chapter 2 and its discussion of death in early nineteenth-century America.

34. Riley, *Sickness, Recovery and Death*, p. 111.

35. Ibid., p. 188.

36. Ibid., p. 192; see also Dorothy P. Rice and Mitchell P. La Plante, "Chronic Illness, Disability, and Increasing Longevity," in Sean Sullivan and Ein Lewin, eds., *The Economics and Ethics of Long-Term Care and Disability* (Washington, D.C.: American Enterprise Institute, 1988), pp. 9–55; Morton Kramer, "The Rising Pandemic of Mental Disorders and Associated Chronic Diseases and Disorders," *Acta Psychiatrica Scandinavica*, suppl. 185, vol. 62 (1980), pp. 382–96; Riley, "Risk of Being Sick," p. 409.

37. Paul Ramsey, *The Patient as Person* (New Haven, Ct.: Yale University Press, 1970), p. 125.

38. I am indebted to Norton Spritz, M.D., for his informative discussions with me about probabilistic judgments in the treatment of the critically ill. See also Robert D. Truog, Allan S. Brett, and Joel Frader, "The Problem with Futility," *New England Journal of Medicine*, vol. 326, no. 23 (June 4, 1992), especially p. 1561.

39. Ariès, *Western Attitudes*, pp. 88–89.

40. See especially Linda L. Emanuel et al., "Advance Directives for Medical Care—a Case for Greater Use," *New England Journal of Medicine*, vol. 324, no. 13 (March 28, 1991), pp. 889–95; David W. Molloy et al., "Treatment Preferences, Attitudes Toward Advance Directives and Concerns About Health Care," *Humane Medicine*, vol. 7, no. 4 (October 1991), pp. 285–90.

41. See, for instance, Michael P. Hosking et al., "Outcomes of Surgery in Patients 90 Years of Age and Older," *Journal of the American Medical Association*, vol. 261, no. 13 (April 9, 1989), pp. 1909–15; Viola B. Latta and Roger E. Keene, "Leading Inpatient Surgical Procedures for Aged Medicare Beneficiaries, 1987," *Health Care Financing Review*, vol. 11, no. 2 (Winter 1989), p. 99–110; L. Henry Edmunds et al., "Open Heart Surgery in Octogenarians," *New England Journal of Medicine*, vol. 319, no. 3 (July 21, 1988), pp. 131–36.

42. See, for example, Marion Danis et al., "Patients and Families' Preferences for Medical Intensive Care," *Journal of the American*

Medical Association, vol. 260, no. 6 (August 12, 1988), pp. 797–802; Nancy R. Zweibel, "Quality of Life Near the End of Life," *Journal of the American Medical Association*, vol. 260, no. 6 (August 12, 1988), pp. 839–40.

43. See Howard Schuman, "Attitudes vs. Actions *Versus* Attitudes vs. Attitudes," *Public Opinion Quarterly*, vol. 36, no. 3 (Fall 1972), pp. 347–54.

44. Dr. Lawrence J. Schneiderman has written that "What happens more often is that physicians take control of decisions, particularly in desperate circumstances, and that patients' prior wishes are unrecognized or ignored" (personal communication).

45. *New York Times*, December 12, 1991, p. 29.

46. Ariès, *Western Attitudes*, p. 107.

47. Sigmund Freud, *The Future of the Illusion* (New York: W. W. Norton, 1989), p. 16.

Chapter 2: *Stripping Death Bare: The Recovery of Nature*

1. Darrel W. Amundsen, "The Physician's Duty to Prolong Life: A Medical Duty Without Classical Roots," *Hasting Center Report*, vol. 8, no. 4 (August 1978), pp. 23–30

2. See Bill McKibben, "The End of Nature," *Earth Ethics*, vol. 1, no. 3 (Spring 1990), pp. 1–8.

3. O. B. Hardison, Jr., *Disappearing Through the Skylight: Culture and Technology in the Twentieth Century* (New York: Viking, 1989), p. 71.

4. Jessica H. Muller and Barbara A. Koenig, "On the Boundary of Life and Death: The Definition of Dying by Medical Residents," in Margaret Lock and Deborah Gordon, eds., *Biomedicine Examined* (Dordrecht: Kluwer Academic Publishers, 1988), p. 369.

5. Hardison, *Disappearing Through the Skylight*, p. xi.

6. See William E. May, "Criteria for Withholding or Withdrawing Treatment," *Linacre Quarterly*, vol. 57, no. 3 (August 1990), pp. 81–90; see also Robert N. Wennberg, *Terminal Choices* (Grand Rapids, Mich.: William B. Eerdmans, 1989), pp. 150 ff.; William E. May, Robert Bally et al., "Feeding and Hydrating the Permanently Unconscious and Other Vulnerable Persons," *Issues in Law and Medicine*, vol. 3, no. 3 (Winter 1987), pp. 203–17.

7. Otto Guttentag, M.D., personal communication. The late Otto

Guttentag was a distinguished professor of medicine at the University of California, San Francisco.

8. The literature on the distinction between killing and allowing to die, or between commission and omission, is enormous. See, for instance, John Harris, "The Marxist Conception of Violence," *Philosophy and Public Affairs*, vol. 3, no. 2 (Winter 1974), pp. 192–220; H. L. A. Hart, "Postscript: Responsibility and Retribution," *Punishment and Responsibility* (New York: Oxford University Press, 1968), pp. 211–30; Daniel Dinello, "On Killing and Letting Die," in Bonnie Steinbock, ed., *Killing and Letting Die* (Englewood Cliffs, N.J.: Prentice-Hall, 1980), pp. 128–31; H. H. Malm, "Killing, Letting Die, and Simple Conflicts," *Philosophy and Public Affairs*, vol. 18, no. 3 (Summer 1989), pp. 238–58; Bonnie Steinbock, "The Intentional Termination of Life," in Steinbock, *Killing and Letting Die*, pp. 245–50; Dan W. Brock, "Taking Human Life," *Ethics*, vol. 95 (July 1985), pp. 851–65; Stanley Hauerwas, "Letting Die or Putting to Death," ch. 10 of Stanley Hauerwas, *Vision and Virtue* (Notre Dame, Ind.: Fides/Claretian, 1974), pp. 166–86; Gail Atkinson, "Killing and Letting Die: Hidden Value Assumptions," *Social Science and Medicine*, vol. 12, no. 23 (1983), pp. 1915–25; James Rachels, *The End of Life* (New York: Oxford University Press, 1986), especially ch. 7 and 8; Helga Kuhse, *The Sanctity-of-Life Doctrine in Medicine: A Critique* (Oxford: Clarendon Press, 1987), especially ch. 2, pp. 31–81.

9. James Rachels, "Active and Passive Euthanasia," *New England Journal of Medicine*, vol. 292, no. 2 (January 9, 1975), p. 79; see also Tom L. Beauchamp, "A Reply to Rachels, on Active and Passive Euthanasia," in Tom L. Beauchamp and Seymour Perlin, eds., *Ethical Issues in Death and Dying* (Englewood Cliffs, N.J.: Prentice-Hall, 1978), pp. 246–58.

10. Rachels, "Active and Passive Euthanasia."

11. See, for instance, Joanne Lynn, ed., *By No Extraordinary Means: The Choice to Forgo Life-Sustaining Food and Water* (Bloomington: Indiana University Press, 1986); Committee for Pro-Life Activities, National Conference of Catholic Bishops, "Nutrition and Hydration: Moral and Pastoral Reflections," Resource Paper (April 1992).

12. H. L. A. Hart and Tony Honoré, *Causation and the Law*, 2nd ed. (Oxford: Clarendon Press, 1989), p. 37.

13. Quoted in Stephen P. Strickland, *Politics, Science, and Dread Disease: A Short History of United States Medical Research Policy* (Cambridge, Mass.: Harvard University Press, 1972), p. 187. Strickland provides an interesting analysis of the struggle between many NIH scientists, who wanted to give priority to basic science and were skeptical of "wars" against disease, and many legislators, lay lobbyists, and medical-advocacy groups, who saw the eradication of disease as the main goal. That struggle has continued to this day, and the victory, I believe, has generally gone to the latter group.

Chapter 3: *The Last Illusion: Regulating Euthanasia*

1. Lord Listowel, in A. B. Downing and Barbara Smoker, eds., *Voluntary Euthanasia* (London: Peter Owen, 1986), p. 6.
2. See especially Robert J. Blendon, Ulrike S. Szalay, and Richard A. Knox, "Should Physicians Aid Their Patients in Dying: The Public Perspective," *Journal of the American Medical Association*, vol. 267, no. 19 (May 20, 1992), pp. 2658–62.
3. Eric J. Cassell, *The Nature of Suffering and the Goals of Medicine* (New York: Oxford University Press, 1991), pp. 34–37; see also David B. Morris, *The Culture of Pain* (Berkeley: University of California Press, 1991); Lana Hartman Landon, "Suffering over Time: Six Varieties of Pain," *Soundings*, vol. 72, no. 1 (Spring 1989), pp. 75–82.
4. See Cassell, *Nature of Suffering*, pp. 103–4.
5. Ibid., especially ch. 3, "The Nature of Suffering," pp. 30–47; Warren Thomas Reich, "Speaking of Suffering: A Moral Account of Compassion," *Soundings*, vol. 72, no. 1 (Spring 1989), pp. 83–108; Stanley Hauerwas, *Suffering Presence* (Notre Dame, Ind.: University of Notre Dame Press, 1986).
6. See Susan James, "The Duty to Relieve Suffering," *Ethics*, vol. 93 (October 1982), pp. 4–21.
7. Hauerwas, *Suffering Presence*, p. 33.
8. Timothy E. Quill, "Death and Dignity: A Case of Individualized Decision Making," *New England Journal of Medicine*, vol. 324, no. 10 (March 7, 1991), p. 693. See also Timothy E. Quill, *Death and Dignity: Making Choices and Taking Charge* (New York: W.W. Norton, 1993).
9. See Judith M. Stillion, Eugene E. McDowell, and Jacque H. May,

Suicide Across the Life Span: Premature Exits (New York: Hemisphere Publishing, 1989), especially ch. 8, pp. 233 ff.

10. *Union Pacific R. Co.* v. *Botsford* (1891), quoted in David W. Meyers, *Medico-Legal Implications of Death and Dying* (Rochester, N.Y.: Lawyers Cooperative Publishing Co., 1981), p. 212.

11. Like many others of late, I have avoided the terms "active euthanasia" and "passive euthanasia." The former was traditionally taken to mean direct killing, and the latter what is now commonly referred to as "allowing to die." I will follow that now common usage, which uses the term "euthanasia" to refer to active killing, and the term "allowing to die" to refer to a situation in which a patient dies of an underlying disease rather than from a human action. I do not believe that there is any significant difference morally between euthanasia and assisted suicide, for two reasons. The first is that assisting in the death of another by supplying that person with the knowledge or material means to commit suicide becomes at least a necessary condition of the death of another. The second reason is that the law in general holds people culpable for actions that are materially responsible for dangerous or lethal outcomes—e.g., providing the gun to be used by another in the pursuit of a crime.

12. John Stuart Mill, "On Liberty," in *Essential Works of John Stuart Mill*, ed. Max Lerner (New York: Bantam Books, 1961), p. 348.

13. Joel Feinberg, "Autonomy, Sovereignty, and Privacy: Moral Ideals in the Constitution?," *Notre Dame Law Review*, vol. 58, no. 3 (February 1983), p. 492; see also Arthur Kuplik, "The Inalienability of Autonomy," *Philosophy and Public Affairs*, vol. 13, no. 4 (Fall 1984), pp. 271–98; Joel Feinberg, "Voluntary Euthanasia and the Inalienable Right to Life," *Philosophy and Public Affairs*, vol. 7, no. 2 (Winter 1978), pp. 93–123.

14. See especially Margaret Pabst Battlin, "Euthanasia," in Donald Van De Veer and Tom Regan, eds., *Health Care Ethics: An Introduction* (Philadelphia: Temple University Press, 1987), pp. 58–97; see also Philippa Foot, "Euthanasia," *Philosophy and Public Affairs*, vol. 6, no. 2 (Winter 1977), pp. 85–112; Institute of Medical Ethics Working Party on the Ethics of Prolonging Life and Assisting Death, "Assisted Death," *Lancet*, vol. 336 (September 8, 1990), pp. 610–13; James Rachels, *The End of Life* (New York: Oxford University Press, 1986); Helga Kuhse, *The Sanctity-of-Life Doctrine*

in Medicine (Oxford: Clarendon Press, 1987); David C. Thomasma and Glenn C. Graber, *Euthanasia: Toward an Ethical Social Policy* (New York: Continuum, 1990); Marvin Kohl, ed., *Beneficent Euthanasia* (Buffalo: Prometheus Books, 1975); Don V. Bailey, *The Challenge of Euthanasia: An Annotated Bibliography on Euthanasia and Related Topics* (Lanham, Md.: University Press of America, 1990); Eike-Henner W. Kluge, *The Ethics of Deliberate Death* (Port Washington, N.Y.: Kennikat Press, 1981).

Courtney Campbell has pointed out to me a trend in the past few years, which was clearly apparent in the 1991 Washington State debate on Initiative 119 (to legalize euthanasia and assisted suicide): proponents of euthanasia placed the stress on self-determination only, with little mention of arguments from mercy. Andrew Greeley has argued, based on data collected by the National Opinion Research Center's annual General Social Survey, that changes in public attitudes on end-of-life issues are "to some extent attributable not to direct change in moral views but to a change in people's tolerance for others' moral views or moral situation" (Andrew Greeley, "Live and Let Die: Changing Attitudes," *Christian Century*, December 4, 1991, p. 1125).

15. Immanuel Kant, "Duties Towards the Body in Regard to Life," in Immanuel Kant, *Lectures on Ethics*, trans. Louis Infield (New York: Harper Torch Books, 1963), p. 148.
16. Maurice A. M. de Wachter, "Euthanasia in the Netherlands," *Hastings Center Report*, vol. 22, no. 2 (March–April 1992), pp. 23–30.
17. See Henk A. M. J. ten Have and Jos V. M. Welie, "Euthanasia: Normal Medical Practice," *Hastings Center Report*, vol. 22, no. 2 (March–April 1992), pp. 34–38. Two recent Dutch studies of euthanasia and other practices concerning the termination of treatment are: "Rapport van de Commissie Onderzoek in Medische Praktijk inzake Euthanasie" [the "Remmelink Report"], *Medische Beslissingen Rond het Levenseinde* (The Hague: Edo Uitgeverij, 1991); and G. van der Wal et al., "Euthanasie en hulp bij zelfdoding," *Medisch Contact*, vol. 46, no. 6 (February 8, 1991), pp. 171–73; the same title continued in the next three issues of the journal. This latter study was translated from the Dutch by the Hemlock Society, "Euthanasia and Assisted Suicide by General Practitioners in the Netherlands," n.d., publication unknown.

18. This conference is summarized in de Wachter, "Euthanasia in the Netherlands"; see another discussion of the conference in Alexander Morgan Capron, "Euthanasia in the Netherlands: American Observations," *Hastings Center Report*, vol. 22, no. 2 (March–April 1992), pp. 30–33.

19. The best accounts of the abuses in the Dutch system are to be found in Carlos F. Gomez, *Regulating Death: Euthanasia and the Case of the Netherlands* (New York: Free Press, 1991); and I. J. Keown, "The Law and Practice of Euthanasia in the Netherlands," *Law Quarterly Review*, January 1992, pp. 51–78; see also John Keown, "On Regulating Death," *Hastings Center Report*, vol. 22, no. 2 (March–April 1992), pp. 39–43.

Chapter 4: Living with the Mortal Self

1. Quoted in Louis A. Ruprecht, Jr., "Nussbaum on Tragedy and the Modern Ethos," *Soundings*, vol. 72, no. 4 (Winter 1989), p. 589. No primary reference is given.

2. William Arrowsmith, "The Criticism of Greek Tragedy," *Tulane Drama Review*, vol. 3, no. 3 (1959), p. 55, quoted in Ruprecht, "Nussbaum on Tragedy," p. 593.

3. Martha C. Nussbaum, *The Fragility of Goodness: Luck and Ethics in Greek Tragedy and Philosophy* (Cambridge: Cambridge University Press, 1986), p. 2.

4. Quoted in Ruprecht, "Nussbaum on Tragedy," p. 589. No primary reference is given.

5. Christopher Lasch, *The True and Only Heaven* (New York: W. W. Norton, 1991), p. 451.

6. Mary Gordon, "The Flight from Women," *New York Times*, June 9, 1991, p. 59.

7. I am indebted to Patrick J. Creevy's superb essay "John Donne's Meditations upon the Magnitude of Disease," *Soundings*, vol. 72, no. 1 (Spring 1989), pp. 61–73, especially pp. 65–66.

8. John Donne, *Devotions upon Emergent Occasions*, ed. Anthony Raspa (New York: Oxford University Press, 1987), p. 7.

9. Ibid., p. 46.

10. Viktor E. Frankl, *Man's Search for Meaning*, trans. Ilse Lasch (New York: Pocket Books, 1963), p. 104.

11. This view is most articulately expressed in Richard Rorty, *Contingency, Irony, and Solidarity* (New York: Cambridge University Press, 1989).
12. Arthur Frank, *At the Will of the Body* (Boston: Houghton Mifflin, 1991), p. 58.
13. Especially helpful here, for accounts of life under the most vicious and oppressive circumstances, are Frankl, *Man's Search for Meaning;* Nathan Sharansky, *Fear No Evil,* trans. Stefani Hoffman (New York: Random House, 1988); Nien Cheng, *Life and Death in Shanghai* (New York: Grove, 1986).
14. Sidney Callahan explores this possibility in *In Good Conscience: Reason and Emotion in Moral Decision Making* (San Francisco: Harper San Francisco, 1991), especially ch. 5.
15. Eric J. Cassell, "The Nature of Suffering and the Goals of Medicine," *New England Journal of Medicine,* vol. 306, no. 11 (March 18, 1982), p. 640.
16. Virginia Woolf, "On Being Ill," in *Collected Essays,* vol. 4 (New York: Harcourt, Brace & World, 1967), p. 194, quoted in Elaine Scarry, *The Body in Pain* (New York: Oxford University Press, 1985), p. 4.
17. Cassell, "Nature of Suffering," p. 642.
18. J. Barry Ferguson, author (with Tom Cowan) of *Living with Flowers* (New York: Rizzoli International, 1990).
19. Department of Health and Human Services, *Aging in America: Trends and Projections* (Washington, D.C.: U.S. Department of Health and Human Services, 1991), p. 117.
20. Leon R. Kass, "Death with Dignity and the Sanctity of Life," in Barry S. Kogan, ed., *A Time to Be Born and a Time to Die* (New York: Aldine DeGruyter, 1991), p. 133.
21. I am indebted to Eric J. Cassell for the distinction between self-mastery and self-control.
22. Michel de Montaigne, "That No Man Should be Called Happy Until After His Death," ch. 19 of "The Essays of Montaigne," in *Essays,* trans. J. M. Cohen (New York: Penguin, 1958), pp. 34–35.
23. Ibid., p. 26.
24. Jeremy Taylor, *The Role and Exercise of Holy Living and Dying* (London: George Rutledge and Sons, 1894), p. 93.

Chapter 5: Nature, Death, and Meaning: Shaping Our End

1. Dylan Thomas, "Do not go gentle into that good night," in *The Collected Poems of Dylan Thomas, 1934–1952* (New York: New Directions, 1971), p. 128. Eva Topinková, M.D., was helpful in discussing with me the problems addressed in this chapter, particularly from the perspective of a different culture.

2. Lewis Thomas, *The Lives of a Cell* (New York: Bantam, 1975), p. 115.

3. See especially Lana Hartman Loudon, "Suffering over Time: Six Varieties of Pain," *Soundings*, vol. 52, no. 2 (Spring 1989), pp. 75–82; David B. Morris, *The Culture of Pain* (Berkeley: University of California Press, 1991).

4. William Hazlitt, "On the Fear of Death," from William Hazlitt, *Table Talk*, quoted in D. J. Enright, ed., *The Oxford Book of Death* (New York: Oxford University Press, 1987), p. 31.

5. See Fred Feldman, "Some Puzzles About the Evil of Death," *Philosophical Review*, vol. 100, no. 2 (April 1991), pp. 205–27.

6. See Gilbert Meilaender's excellent essay "Mortality: The Measure of Our Days," *First Things*, February 1991, pp. 14–21; Meilaender perceptively compares E. B. White's views on mortality in *Charlotte's Web*, Felix Salten's in *Bambi*, and C. S. Lewis' in *The Last Battle*.

7. Some fine articles on this subject can be found in Steven Sanders and David R. Cheney, eds., *The Meaning of Life* (Englewood Cliffs, N.J.: Prentice-Hall, 1980).

8. I am adapting here, by adding a third ingredient, the distinctions advanced by Irving Singer in *Meaning in Life: The Creation of Value* (New York: Free Press, 1992), p. 23.

9. Arthur C. McGill, *Death and Life: An American Theology* (Philadelphia: Fortress Press, 1987), pp. 9–10.

10. Jean-Paul Sartre, *Being and Nothingness*, trans. Hazel E. Barnes (New York: Washington Square Press, 1966), pp. 682–83.

11. Thomas Nagel, *Mortal Questions* (Cambridge: Cambridge University Press, 1979), p. 10.

12. McGill, *Death and Life*, pp. 11–12.

13. Ibid., p. 12.

14. Jeremy Taylor, *The Golden Grove: Selected Passages from the Sermons*

and Writings of Jeremy Taylor (London: Oxford University Press, 1930), p. 257.

15. Hans Jonas, "The Burden and Blessing of Mortality," *Hastings Center Report*, vol. 22, no. 1 (January–February 1992), p. 34.

16. Ibid., p. 37.

17. Ibid., p. 39.

18. Singer, *Meaning in Life*, pp. 58–59.

19. Ibid., p. 60.

20. George Santayana, "A Long Way Round to Nirvana; or Much Ado About Dying," in *Some Turns of Thought in Modern Philosophy: Five Essays* (New York: Charles Scribner's Sons, 1933), pp. 98–101, quoted in Singer, *Meaning in Life*, p. 51.

21. Paul Ramsey, "The Indignity of 'Death with Dignity,' " *Hastings Center Studies*, vol. 2, no. 2 (May 1974), pp. 50, 52.

22. Ibid., p. 62. See also Gilbert Meilaender, " 'Love's Casuistry': Paul Ramsey on Caring for the Terminally Ill," *Journal of Religious Ethics*, Fall 1991, pp. 133–56.

Chapter 6: Pursuing a Peaceful Death

1. James R. Wyngaarden, Lloyd H. Smith, and J. Claude Bennett, eds., *Cecil Textbook of Medicine*, 19th ed. (Philadelphia: W. B. Saunders, 1992).

2. Richard W. Momeyer, *Confronting Death* (Bloomington: Indiana University Press, 1988), p. 28.

3. See Robert F. Weir and Larry Gostin, "Decisions to Abate Life-Sustaining Treatment for Nonautonomous Patients," *Journal of the American Medical Association*, vol. 264, no. 14 (October 10, 1990), pp. 1846–53.

4. For a valuable discussion of the problems and possibilities here, see M. Pabst Battin, "The Least Worst Death," *Hastings Center Report*, vol. 13, no. 2 (April 1983), pp. 13–16.

5. These ideas are developed at greater length in my book *What Kind of Life: The Limits of Medical Progress* (New York: Simon & Schuster, 1990), pp. 135–57.

6. Leon R. Kass, *Toward a More Natural Science: Biology and Human Affairs* (New York: Free Press, 1985), p. 162.

7. The Loran Commission, *Making Difficult Health Care Decisions*, vol.

I—*The National Survey* (New York: Louis Harris and Associates, 1987), p. 25.

8. See Lawrence J. Schneiderman, Nancy S. Jecker, and Albert R. Jonsen, "Medical Futility: Its Meaning and Ethical Implications," *Annals of Internal Medicine*, vol. 112, no. 12 (June 15, 1990), pp. 949–54; John D. Lantos et al., "The Illusion of Futility in Medical Practice," *American Journal of Medicine*, vol. 87 (July 1989), pp. 81–84; Tom Tomlinson and Howard Brody, "Futility and the Ethics of Resuscitation," *Journal of the American Medical Association*, vol. 264, no. 10 (September 12, 1990), pp. 1276–80; Stuart J. Youngner, "Who Defines Futility?," *Journal of the American Medical Association*, vol. 260, no. 14 (October 14, 1988), pp. 2094–95.

9. See Daniel Callahan, "Medical Futility, Medical Necessity: The Problem-Without-a-Name," *Hastings Center Report*, vol. 21, no. 4 (July–August 1991), pp. 30–35.

Chapter 7: Watching and Waiting

1. I found John Bowker's discussion of this theme illuminating in his book *The Meanings of Death* (Cambridge: Cambridge University Press, 1991), pp. 31 ff.

2. Simone de Beauvoir, *A Very Easy Death* (London: Weidenfeld, 1966), p. 106, quoted in Bowker, *Meanings of Death*.

3. James J. Farrell, *Inventing the American Way of Death, 1830–1920* (Philadelphia: Temple University Press, 1980), pp. 216, 221.

4. Bowker, *Meanings of Death*, p. 211.

INDEX